江苏省十四五教育科学规划2022年度省重点课题（编号B/2022/01/79）

新医科学科英语导学

主　编　朱春梅

副主编　朱九扬　刘　冰

李洪民　吴震宇

U0250618

南京大学出版社

图书在版编目(CIP)数据

新医科学科英语导学 / 朱春梅主编. — 南京 : 南京
大学出版社,2024.8
(学科英语系列丛书 / 钟家宝主编)
ISBN 978 - 7 - 305 - 27074 - 1

Ⅰ.①新… Ⅱ.①朱… Ⅲ.①医学 – 英语 –
高等学校 – 教材 Ⅳ.①R

中国国家版本馆 CIP 数据核字(2023)第 100540 号

出版发行 南京大学出版社
社　　址 南京市汉口路 22 号　　　邮　编　210093
丛 书 名 学科英语系列丛书
丛书主编 钟家宝
书　　名 新医科学科英语导学
　　　　　XINYIKE XUEKE YINGYU DAOXUE
主　　编 朱春梅
责任编辑 张淑文
照　　排 南京开卷文化传媒有限公司
印　　刷 南京百花彩色印刷广告制作有限责任公司
开　　本 787 mm×1092 mm　1/16 开　印张 12.5　字数 405 千
版　　次 2024 年 8 月第 1 版　2024 年 8 月第 1 次印刷
ISBN 978 - 7 - 305 - 27074 - 1

定　　价 50.00 元
网　　址:http://www.njupco.com
官方微博:http://weibo.com/njupco
微信服务号:njuyuexue
销售咨询热线:(025)83594756

Contents

Unit 1
Precision Medicine

Guiding to learn

The concept of precision medicine (sometimes called personalized medicine, genomic medicine, or precision oncology) was developed in the early 21st century with the overall goal of tailoring tumor treatment for each patient to achieve higher efficacy of clinical outcomes. Precision medicine is an evolving treatment method that diagnoses, treats, and prevents cancer using genomic information from patients' tumor. Although precision medicine has traditionally relied on the genomic analysis to identify mutational targetable cancer cell, the majority of identified tumor specific molecular targets has not been recommended or only in silico predicted effect on the corresponding protein, and the field of molecular analysis has evolved to include additional analysis techniques such as RNA sequencing, proteomics, or metabolomics.

Discuss the following questions with your partners.

1. What is precision medicine?
2. What is precision medicine's main concern?
3. What is next-generation sequencing?

Task 1　Learn the following general academic vocabulary.

analyse assessment derivation indicateindividual variability positive potential previously relevant strategy exclusive framework illustrate layer outcome sequence validate annual integrate investigate mechanism overall statistical status subsequently evolve external perspective precise stability accurate domain furthermore incorporate reveal underlying comprehensive unique clarify fluctuation highlight induce

Beginning to read

Task 2   Now read the text.

Text A

What Is Precision Medicine?
I. R. König et al

1. The term "precision medicine"（精准医学）has become very popular in recent years, fuelled by scientific as well as political perspectives. It has superseded the term "personalised medicine"（个性化治疗）, which was defined synonymously, but then dismissed wi10th the argument that physicians have always treated patients on a personalised level. Indeed, the personal approach that is an inherent part of the doctor-patient relationship is a central aspect of precision medicine, but is not a new invention. However, new biomedical information might add substantial information beyond signs and symptoms that were previously observable, and the term precision medicine implies the novelty of this concept, which is the incorporation of a wide array of individual data, including clinical, lifestyle, genetic and further biomarker information.

2. A successful example that is frequently cited in this respect is the determination of the human epidermal growth factor receptor（HER）- 2（人表皮生长因子受体- 2）status in breast cancer patients. Initially, HER - 2 was discovered to be a prognostic factor（预后因素）with positive patients having a higher probability of a more aggressive course of disease. Subsequently, clinical trials showed the efficacy of the monoclonal antibody trastuzumab, which is directed against an epitope on the external domain of the HER - 2 protein; now, trastuzumab is given only to the subgroup of HER - 2 - positive females, thus proving the gain of including gene expression data. Examples of cases of obstructive airway diseases are shown in Table 1, which summarises phenotyping of individuals based on different investigational approaches.

3. Despite the obvious success of this and other examples, the meaning of precision medicine, and how it is related to or different from other popular terms such as "stratified medicine"（分层医学）, "targeted therapy"（靶向治疗）or deep phenotyping remains unclear. Commonly used definitions of precision medicine include the following aspects. 1) Focus on result, i.e. personalised treatment strategies; some define precision medicine as "treatments targeted to the needs of individual patients on

the basis of genetic, biomarker, phenotypic or psychosocial characteristics that distinguish a given patient from other patients with similar clinical presentations". 2) Focus on process and utilised data: others emphasise the data by describing precision medicine as a model that integrates clinical and other data to stratify patients into novel subgroups; it is hoped that these have a common basis of disease susceptibility and manifestation and thus potentially allow for more precise therapeutic solutions.

4. Thus, the focus of commonly applied definitions is on the stratification of patients, sometimes referred to as a novel taxonomy, and this is derived using large-scale data that go beyond the classical "signs-and-symptoms"（体征与症状）approach. Finding this novel taxonomy has been described as identifying "treatable traits", i.e. disease subgroups that can be treated in a better way because of more precise and validated phenotypic recognition（表型识别）or due to a better understanding of the critical causal pathways.

5. While these aspects are relevant, this description of precision medicine leaves open a number of questions, such as 1) how can or cannot precision medicine be distinguished from other related terms; 2) when does precision medicine actually begin; 3) what are the target achievements and underlying concepts of the idea of precision medicine; 4) how does the stratification of patients translate into better healthcare; 5) can precision medicine really be viewed as the end-point of a novel stratification of patients, as implied, or is it rather a greater whole.

6. To clarify this, the aim of this article is to provide a more comprehensive definition that focuses on precision medicine as a process. It will be shown that this proposed framework incorporates the derivation of novel taxonomies and their role in healthcare as part of the cycle, but also covers related terms.

7. Obviously, precision medicine is not an exclusive need or a unique feature of respiratory medicine. However, asthma and chronic obstructive pulmonary disease (COPD)（慢性阻塞性肺疾病）are the most common chronic diseases worldwide, with increasing prevalence, mortality and morbidity. Specifically, the Global Burden of Disease Study presented rankings for years lived with disability, among which asthma ranked 14th and COPD ranked 5th in 2010. The annual costs of healthcare and lost productivity in the European Union due to COPD are estimated to be €48.4 billion per year and those due to asthma to be €33.9 billion per year. These data highlight the need for optimal management of the most prevalent chronic respiratory diseases, and we therefore focus on asthma and COPD to illustrate the meaning of precision medicine.

8. In our framework, precision medicine is defined as a process which is depicted in figure 1 and described further in the following sections. The concept incorporates the following ideas: 1) as the process includes a number of feedback loops, there is no steady end-point of precision medicine where, finally, precise medical care is provided

to the patients; 2) the cycle implies that there are ongoing efforts to become ever more precise; 3) finer and more accurate stratifications of patients can be interim results of the overall process, which is captured by the term "stratified medicine".

9. An important aspect of this framework therefore is that data assessed in the patients are used to try to develop clinically relevant models, and that the results of these analyses then inform the further assessment of patients, thus emphasising the definition of a process and precision medicine as an evolving result.

10. Whereas the question of how and which patients are recruited, i.e. the study design, therefore depends on the specific research question, the characterising feature in this process is the nature of information gathered in these patients. Specifically, the novel taxonomy aimed for in precision medicine does not rely on the classical signs-and-symptoms approach, but adds data from other sources, such as gene expression analyses.

11. As an example, asthma is known to be a heterogeneous disease with variation in the degree and type of airway inflammation. To investigate the underlying molecular mechanisms, WOODRUFF et al. performed a genome-wide gene expression analysis comparing the expression between subjects with asthma, nonasthmatic smokers and healthy controls. They identified three genes as highly induced in airway epithelial cells from subjects with asthma, namely POSTN (periostin), CLCA2 (chloride channel, calcium-activated, family member 1) and SERPINB2 (serine peptidase inhibitor, clade B, member 2). Furthermore, interleukin (IL)- 13 as a key indicator of T-helper type 2 (Th2) inflammation in asthma was found to directly induce the expression of these genes in epithelial cells in vitro. The authors postulated that these genes can be viewed as biomarkers of classic IL－13－driven asthma. These data suggest that expression levels in these genes can be considered as part of the data profile of asthma patients.

12. Further examples illustrating that comprehensive molecular analysis is increasingly being used routinely derive from the Unbiased Biomarkers in Prediction of Respiratory Disease Outcomes (U-BIOPRED)(预测呼吸系统疾病预后的无偏倚生物标志物) project, which aims to elucidate the mechanisms and biological pathways of severe asthma. In this cohort, KUO et al. identified three TACs(转录组相关簇) by analysing sputum cell transcriptomics(转录组学) from moderate-to-severe asthmatic subjects and healthy controls. TAC1 comprises an IL－13/Th2－high predominantly eosinophilic cluster, while TAC2 and TAC3 are non-Th2 phenotypes. Eosinophilic asthma was predominantly associated with TAC1, but also present in TAC3, whereas neutrophilic asthma was mainly present with TAC2. Of note, previously used biomarkers such as exhaled nitric oxide and periostin were no different in the three TACs. Cluster analysis of differentially expressed genes defined subgroups among the severe asthmatics that differed in molecular responses to oral corticosteroids(皮质类固

醇). This approach might identify molecular pathways for further studies in poorly controlled asthmatics.

From European Respiratory Journal，2017，50(4)

New words and expressions

epidermal /ˌepɪˈdɜːməl/ *adj*. of or relating to a cuticle or cuticula 表皮的；外皮的

diagnostic /ˌdaɪəɡˈnɒstɪk/ *adj*. a diagnostic clinic，a diagnostic reading test，diagnostic information，or a diagnostic sign of yellow fever，diagnostic information 诊断的，判断的；(因症状特异而)能指示某种疾病性质的；(生物学上的某一物种、属类或现象所)特有的

prognostic /prɒɡˈnɒstɪk/ *adj*. of or relating to prediction；having value for making predictions 预后的；预兆的

monoclonal /ˌmɒnəʊˈkləʊnəl/ *adj*. forming or derived from a single clone 单克隆的；单细胞繁殖的

trastuzumab /trɑːstˈjuːzjuːmæb/ *n*. 曲妥珠单抗(抗肿瘤药)

susceptibility /səˌseptəˈbɪləti/ *n*. the state of being susceptible very likely to be influenced or easily affected by sth 易受影响(或伤害等)的特性；感情脆弱之处，情感的要害(susceptibilities)

phenotype /ˈfiːnətaɪp/ *n*. the set of characteristics of a living thing, resulting from its combination of genes and the effect of its environment 表型，表现型(基因和环境作用的结合而形成的一组生物特征)

manifestation /ˌmænɪfeˈsteɪʃ(ə)n/ *n*. an event，action or thing that is a sign that sth exists or is happening；the act of appearing as a sign that sth exists or is happening 显示；表明；表示

chronic /ˈkrɒnɪk/ *adj*. (especially of a disease) lasting for a long time；difficult to cure or get rid of，or having had a disease for a long time 长期的；慢性的；难以治愈(或根除)的；长期患病的

heterogeneous /ˌhetərəˈdʒiːnɪəs/ *adj*. consisting of many different kinds of people or things 由很多种类组成的；各种各样的

asthma /ˈæsmə/ *n*. a medical condition of the chest that makes breathing difficult 气喘；哮喘

inflammation /ˌɪnfləˈmeɪʃn/ *n*. a condition in which a part of the body becomes red，sore and swollen because of infection or injury 发炎；炎症

transcriptome /trænˈskrɪptəʊm/ *n*. a collection of all the messenger RNA in a particular cell 转录组

transcriptomics /trænˈskrɪptəʊmɪks/ *n*. 转录组学

interleukin /ɪnˈtəlʊkɪn/ *n*. a substance extracted from white blood cells that stimulates their activity against infection and may be used to combat some forms of cancer 白

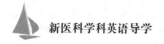

细胞介素

pathomechanism /pæˈθəʊmɪkənɪzəm/ *n*. 病理机理,病理(学)机制

eosinophilic /ˌiːəsɪˈnɒfɪlɪk/ *adj*. of or relating to eosinophil 嗜曙红的,嗜酸性的;嗜曙红细胞的

After reading

Task 3　Read Text A again and answer the following questions.

1. How much do you know about precision medicine?

2. What is the authors' framework of precision medicine?

Task 4　Check your vocabulary. Fill in the blanks with the correct form of the words from the following box, each word can be used only once.

arbitrary(*adj*.)　assign(*v*.)　context(*n*.)　criterion(*n*.)　data(*n*.)　denote(*v*.) devise(*v*.)　formulate(*v*.)　ignore(*v*.)　impact(*n*.)　similar(*adj*.)　summary(*n*.) usage(*n*.)　vertical(*adj*.)

1. Metasurfaces have been widely studied for _____ manipulation of the amplitude, phase and polarization of a field at the sub-wavelength scale.

2. These differences among individuals highlight the importance of considering the traits of dispersers in the _____ in which they are moving.

3. The _____ dashed line indicates the time depth of the parasite tree.

4. We found that the program could confidently _____ fragments in very incomplete data.

5. Diagnosis was classically based on presence of at least two out of three "majors" _____ of Whitaker's triad (candidiasis, autoimmune hypoparathyroidism and adrenal insufficiency).

6. The authors of a previous study proposed a statistically based approach to _____ treatment outcome, translating pretest and posttest scores into clinically relevant categories, such as recovery and reliable improvement.

7. Here is some _____ to help provide some perspectives on these questions.

8. We can _____ biotechnological or genetic techniques to promote plant survival in the stressful conditions.

9. This first part discusses various materials used to _____ microcapsules, such as the three encapsulating polymers as well as protective colloids, plasticizers and surfactants.

10. Biofuels must be combined with robust, truly renewable energy sources that are not agriculturally based to lessen the _____ on global biodiversity.

Task 5   Build your vocabulary. Read the sentences below, decide which word in each bracket is more suitable.

1. It is increasingly (evident/visible) that the relevant ecologies are both those encountered within hosts and in host populations, manifested as adaptive immune responses.

2. Peer reviewed biomedical journals are expected to (make/publish) accurate and important information.

3. (Involving/Including) patient partners improves research processes, outcomes, and translating findings into practice. Two alternative tectonic reconstructions a land connection between the Greater Antilles and either mainland South America or Central America will be discussed.

4. In addition, the advent of immunotherapy over recent years has dramatically changed the (negative/bleak) outcomes observed in malignancies such as melanoma.

5. After understanding the (environment/ecology)of plague, preventative and control measures at each stage of the infectious cycle and their effectiveness are examined.

6. In order to (evaluate/judge) commonly used pain intensity measures, 75 chronic pain patients were asked to rate 4 kinds of pain (present, least, most, and average) using 6 scales.

7. We tested whether individual bettongs could adjust home (range/variety) size to maintain access to essential habitat across three sites differing in degree of fragmentation.

8. Children in joint physical or legal custody were better (modified /adjusted) than children in sole-custody settings, but no different from those in intact families.

9. With the annealing temperature below a critical value, the bandwidth of Bragg gratings induced by Type I-IR and Type II-IR index change was (restricted/narrowed) without the reduction of reflectivity.

10. To (acquire/derive) calcium content weight fraction from microCT scans, a measure of tissue density is required and a constant value is traditionally used.

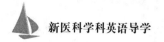

Guiding to learn

Task 6   Learn the following general academic vocabulary.

analysis area available constitute majority process theoretically categorized conduct impact positive range regulatory component emphasize technique access contrast emerge implementation expansion generate domain initiative nevertheless utilization isolation phenomena publication detect inevitably manipulate unbiased portion

Beginning to read

Task 7   Now read the text.

Text B

Recent Major Transcriptomics and Epitranscriptomics Contributions toward Personalized and Precision Medicine
Ghada Mubarak & Farah R. Zahir

1. Since microarray（微阵列）technology heralded the advent of the third era in medical diagnostics in the early "noughties", clinical medical genetics has focused on genome-wide screens rather than targeted approaches. Shortly after chromosomal microarray analysis（CMA）（染色体微阵列分析）was accepted and widely adopted as a first-tier diagnostic test in medical genetics, next generation sequencing（NGS）（新一代测序）technologies exploded onto the scene. Indeed, the past decade has seen an acceleration in the development and implementation of a plethora of NGS based genomics screens that are ever-decreasing in cost, ever-increasing in diagnostic and clinical utility, and therefore, unsurprisingly, undergoing rapid expansion in utilization by diagnostic laboratories. The most common NGS screens involve interrogating the DNA sequence of the protein coding portion of the genome, termed whole exome sequencing（WES）（全外显子组测序）, followed by interrogating the entire whole genome, termed whole genome sequencing（WGS）. These techniques and

their reach in medical diagnostics have been extensively reported on and reviewed.

2. The latter half of the past decade, however, has given us a wide range of NGS-based screening methods other than WES and WGS. The variety and frequency of publication on the plethora of such "omics"（组学）approaches admittedly have even caused amusement as scientists and health care providers grapple to keep abreast of them. Indeed, tropes such as "other-omics" or "everything-omics" have commanded some popularity in various media. Nevertheless, some of these "other-omics" have come into their own as robust sciences that are now moving inevitably and one hopes, with very positive contribution, into the sphere of the clinic.

3. In this paper, we overview the most relevant contributions of a major omics discipline-transcriptomics, and briefly touch on its continuum—epitranscriptomics（表观转录组学）—toward efforts in disease characterization and diagnostics as part of personalized and precision medicine initiatives. We focus our review on major advances in trascriptomics（转录组学）for three diseases: cancer, cardiovascular disease（CVD）（心血管学病）, and neurodevelopmental disorders（NDDs）（神经发育障碍）. They constitute the three disease areas where, in our estimation, the most significant developments in precision and/or personalized medicine have occurred. The recently emerging field of epitranscriptomics is necessarily dependent on the field of transcriptomics. Epitranscriptomics is the study of epi-modifications, i.e., chemical changes to the expressed gene transcript. Thus, advances in this field are intrinsically tied to advances in transcriptomics research. When considered via the lens of precision or personalized medicine, therefore of the three diseases we discuss for transcriptomics advances, we find the most notable contributions are in the ND domain. Hence, we only discuss epitranscriptomics for ND in depth.

Transcriptomics—A Key "Other-Ome": An Introduction and Overview

Defining the "Ome"

4. Firstly, we must emphasize that when using the term "omic", what is intended is that the whole is looked at rather than a part or a target. While there are reports that the first coining of the term "genomics"（基因组学）occurred in 1986 by Dr. Thomas Roderick during an informal meeting, the word "genome" was first reported in 1920 in a German publication by Hans Winkler, who stated "I propose the expression Genom for the haploid chromosome set, which, together with the pertinent protoplasm, specifies the material foundations of the species . . .". From this, was birthed the phenomena of terming every possible biological science where the whole is looked at as "something or the other-ome"! In fact, so ubiquitous was the trend at one time, that an interesting report speculates on the connection of this sound to a mantra invoking the divine. It should also be noted, that while it may sound as if the suffix "ome" has a Greek origin, no such reports exist. Nevertheless, the suffix has claimed as

新医科学科英语导学

foundational a place as other medical terms with origin in the ancient Greek medical lexicon. Indeed，rightly so，as the immense impact of "omics" science and clinical contributions to society in numerous ways testify.

Transcriptomes and Transcriptomics

5. While the study of the whole complement of DNA sequence has been well established in personalized medicine, especially WES and WGS, transcriptomics(转录组学) is slowly but surely catching up. Transcriptomics refers to the study of the full complement of gene expression. This can be understood as the sum of the mRNAs in a cell or sample. However, the major point to note is that the transcriptome(转录组) includes all the product of transcription, sans inherent consideration of subsequent translation. In other words, while one can select only the mRNA for analysis, the transcriptome theoretically includes all types of RNAs produced. The vast majority of these are not mRNA. They include a diverse array of RNAs, collectively termed non-coding RNA (ncRNA), comprising several major RNA classes such as ribosomal(核糖体的) RNA (rRNA), transfer RNA (tRNA), long non-coding RNA (lncRNA), micro-RNA (miRNA), etc. The above ncRNAs may be categorized in several ways, a useful grouping involves rRNAs and tRNAs together being termed "housekeeping RNAs", while the other ncRNA classes are included in "regulatory RNAs" when it has been proven they are involved in cellular regulatory processes.

6. The vast majority of the ncRNA pool is rRNA, which a cell produces in copious amounts as it forms the building material for ribosomes. rRNA from an isolate is generally depleted prior to sequencing as their abundance seriously impedes detecting signal from other RNAs, especially if mRNA is the objective of the assay. However, there are many classes of ncRNA other than rRNA, and they have recently been found to play an essential role in regulation of transcription, as we elaborate on below. For a full review of all rRNA classes see.

7. Of the entire human genome, only $\sim 2\%$ is considered to be protein-coding gene sequence(蛋白质编码基因序列). However, $\sim 70{-}80\%$ of the genome is transcribed. If one supposes that about half of protein-coding genes(蛋白质基因编码) were to be transcribed in a given cell, and that 80% of the genome was represented in that cell's transcriptome at a given time, fully 98.75% of the total transcripts are in fact ncRNA. Thus, while a transcriptomic assay is able to capture the entire complement of transcribed sequence, it remains up to the study design to determine which RNA component will be analyzed. Several transcriptomic studies are limited to mRNA alone, often loosely termed "gene expression"(基因表达)analysis. However, others include specific RNA classes, such as lncRNA, sncRNA, miRNA, as examples. Therefore, while it is established that the transcriptome is a capture of RNA sequence, it is important that definitions are examined carefully when speaking of transcriptomes or transcriptomic profiling.

10

Gene Expression Arrays

8. The earliest transcriptomic assay was a complement to the earliest genomic assay(基因组分析)—the microarray. Soon after the first successful CMA genomics screens（基因组学筛选）were conducted，it did not take long to demonstrate CMA for the coding transcriptome，by simply manipulating an mRNA sample to convert it back to cDNA and using the same techniques as for genomic CMA. The earliest reported gene expression array studies utilized this approach. As microarray technology became more mainstream，all the major microarray providers developed and marketed specialized microarray platforms for gene expression studies. Illumina®，so well known for their NGS（next generation sequencing）sequencers，also entered the expression microarray field with its still popular Illumina BeadArray™ microarray. Notably，all the above platforms are configured by default to mRNA expression analysis，as the technology is limited by only being able to interrogate products which will hybridize（杂交）a pre-existing probe sequence manufactured and bonded to the microarray. Thus，in order to detect an expression signal，the sequence being looked for must already be known，and therefore，this meant that only mRNA was typically included.

From Journal of Personalized Medicine，*2022*，*12（199）*

After reading

Task 8　Build your vocabulary.

Directions：Match the following words with their corresponding definitions and Chinese equivalents.

English：microarray　plethora　genomics　positive　continuum　intrinsical　speculate　ubiquitous

Chinese：基因组学　微阵列芯片　积极乐观的　本质的　过剩　连续统　普遍存在的　猜测

Paras. 1—4

English	Chinese	Definition
1. _____	_____	a. characterized by or displaying affirmation or acceptance or certainty etc.
2. _____	_____	b. a multiplex lab-on-a-chip
3. _____	_____	c. a continuous nonspatial whole or extent or succession in which no part or portion is distinct of distinguishable from adjacent parts

4. _____ _____   d. belonging to a thing by its very nature

5. _____ _____   e. the branch of genetics that studies organisms in terms of their genomes（their full DNA sequences）

6. _____ _____   f. an amount that is greater than is needed or can be used

7. _____ _____   g. seeming to be everywhere or in several places at the same time；very common

8. _____ _____   h. to form an opinion about sth without knowing all the details or facts

Paras. 5—9

English：transcriptome cellular copious essential elaborate hybridization sequence

Chinese：详尽的 充裕的 细胞的 转录组 必不可少的 次序 杂交

English	**Chinese**	**Definition**

9. _____ _____   i. very complicated and detailed；carefully prepared and organized

10. _____ _____   j. a collection of all the messenger RNA in a particular cell

11. _____ _____   k. completely necessary；extremely important in a particular situation or for a particular activity

12. _____ _____   l. connected with or consisting of the cells of plants or animals

13. _____ _____   m. in large amounts

14. _____ _____   n. the order that events，actions，etc. happen in or should happen in

15. _____ _____   o. (genetics) the act of mixing different species or varieties of animals or plants and thus to produce hybrids

Guiding to learn

Task 9 Learn the following general academic vocabulary from the word bank.

option mediate implicate incidence traditional illustrate complexity highlight contribute potential identify alteration guideline variability achieve emergence investigator technology previously implication significantly initiate comprehensive expand validate reveal demonstrate utilize paradigm conventional

Beginning to read

Task 10　Now read the text.

Text C

Current Trends in Precision Medicine and Next-Generation Sequencing in Head and Neck Cancer
Roberto N. Solis et al

1. Despite substantial advances in imaging, diagnostics, and treatment options for patients with head and neck squamous cell carcinoma (HNSCC)(头颈部鳞状细胞癌), 5-year overall survival (OS) has only modestly improved in the last few decades. In 2021, it is estimated that 14,620 deaths will occur in the USA due to HNSCC alone. This disease has largely been an environmentally mediated malignancy with tobacco and alcohol being the most important drivers of carcinogenesis. Currently, the mainstay treatment for HNSCC remains nonselective therapies with a combination of surgery, radiotherapy, and cytotoxic chemotherapy options.

2. In recent years, new epidemiologic patterns have arisen in HNSCC patients. The human papillomavirus (HPV)(人乳头瘤病毒) has been implicated in the rise of incidence for oropharyngeal SCC, with more favorable survival outcomes compared to HPV-negative disease. Additionally, there has been a rise in incidence of oral cavity SCC in younger patients that lack the traditional risk factors demonstrating a possibly distinct clinical and histopathologic(组织病理学) entity. Despite using traditional factors to help predict outcomes (namely tumor stage), we are realizing that not all HNSCC behaves the same, with subsets of HNSCC having better or worse outcomes than predicted by current staging algorithms. Combined, these findings highlight the critical need for further analysis of factors contributing to HNSCC carcinogenesis and prognosis. Key among these is incorporating precision medicine into care, including the validation of prognostic biomarkers and development of patient-specific treatment regimens.

3. Next-generation sequencing (NGS) has unlocked the potential to explore the molecular aspects of HNSCC with an aim to enhance precision medicine. Included in these goals for NGS are to highlight prognostic molecular alterations as well as to identify actionable genomic alterations for a variety of cancers, including HNSCC. While NGS has gained popularity among oncologists, it remains in its infancy, and

currently there are no evidence-based guidelines to guide our use of NGS clinically.

4. In the field of head and neck cancer，historical success with precision medicine has been limited. Despite the growing interest and efforts in exploring novel therapeutics，cetuximab（西妥昔单抗）（an anti-EGFR antibody）remains the only FDA-approved targeted therapeutic agent for HNSCC. The plentitude of mutations，heterogeneity（异质性），and variability in HNSCC pose challenges in designing a single "magic bullet"（灵丹妙药）agent，and therefore，patients currently require multimodal therapy to achieve optimal outcomes. Herein，we review the current state of clinical investigations in precision medicine，targeted therapies，and NGS in HNSCC. Additionally，we discuss the most recent advances，the opportunities，and gaps in knowledge related to the emergence of precision medicine within the field.

5. When imatinib（伊马替尼）entered the market as a "miracle drug"（仙丹妙药）for the treatment of chronic myelogenous leukemia（慢性髓细胞性白血病），the world was excited for the untapped potential of precision medicine and targeted therapies in all cancers. Within the field of head and neck cancer，there was early optimism as investigators identified potential genetic targets that were impacting oncologic prognosis such as EGFR and BCL2. While these discoveries were promising，NGS technology was in its infancy to validate findings in larger cohorts and to perform genetic screens in large scales. Two landmark papers，published sequentially in 2011，provided the framework for understanding the landscape of mutations in HNSCC through whole exome sequencing. In addition to the previously identified genes implicated in HNSCC，Stransky et al. discovered that at least 30% of cases harbored mutations that regulate squamous differentiation. Agrawal et al. had similar findings in their cohort and also elucidated that 89% of HPV-negative tumors had mutations in tumor suppressor genes，with challenging implications on targeted therapy options. Consistent with epidemiologic studies suggestive of biologic differences，HPV-positive tumors had significantly less mutational burden overall，and none harbored TP53 mutations.

6. In 2006，The Cancer Genome Atlas（TCGA）（癌症基因组图谱）project was initiated to further advance our understanding of cancer genomics. This program has amassed thousands of high-quality cancer samples that have been characterized and have allowed for the research community to develop novel cancer therapeutics. In 2015，the TCGA published the most comprehensive integrative genomic analysis of HNSCC in 279 patients，which expanded our understanding of the mutational landscape of HNSCC. HPV-positive tumors were characterized by a loss of TRAF3，activating mutations of PIK3CA，and amplification of E2F1，while HPV-negative tumors mainly had TP53 mutations. In a subset of HPV-negative tumors that behaved more favorably，they expressed normal TP53，but mutations in CASP8 and HRAS. They also discovered CCND1 to be amplified in about one-third of HNSCC. Notably，

there are some limitations with existing genomic studies，as outlined below.

7. Recently，a multicenter consortium characterized the somatic mutational landscape of 227 oral tongue SCCs and identified two additional novel driver genes，in addition to validating previously identified mutations. Analysis of 107 patients that were early onset (< 50 years of age) revealed significantly fewer non-silent mutations independent of smoking status，with implications that early onset oral tongue SCC may be a distinct subtype of HNSCC.

From Current Treatment Options in Oncology，2022，23(2)

New words and expressions

malignancy /məˈlɪgnənsi/ *n*. a malignant mass of tissue，in the body the state of being malignant 恶性肿瘤，恶性

carcinogenesis /ˌkɑːsɪnəʊˈdʒenɪsɪs/ *n*. the development of cancerous cells from normal ones 致癌作用

epidemiologic /ˈepɪˌdiːmɪəˈlɒdʒɪk/ *adj*. of or relating to epidemiology 流行病学的；传染病学的

regimen /ˈredʒɪmən/ *n*. (also regime) a set of rules about food and exercise or medical treatment that you follow in order to stay healthy or to improve your health 生活规则；养生之道；养生法

oncology /ɒŋˈkɒlədʒi/ *n*. the scientific study of and treatment of tumours in the body 肿瘤学

therapy /ˈθerəpi/ *n*. (pl. -ies) the treatment of a physical problem or an illness 治疗；疗法

mutation /mjuːˈteɪʃn/ *n*. a process in which the genetic material of a person，a plant or an animal changes in structure when it is passed on to children，etc.，causing different physical characteristics to develop；a change of this kind (生物物种的) 变异，突变

amplification /ˌæmplɪfɪˈkeɪʃn/ *n*. a usually massive replication of genetic material and especially of a gene or DNA sequence 扩大，增强；扩增

actionable /ˈækʃənəbl/ *adj*. capable of being acted on 可操作的；可执行的；可行动的

randomize /ˈrændəmaɪz/ *v*. to use a method in an experiment，a piece of research，etc. that gives every item an equal chance of being considered；to put things in a random order 使随机化；(使)作任意排列

cytotoxic /ˌsaɪtəʊˈtɒksɪk/ *adj*. poisonous to living cells；denoting certain drugs used in the treatment of leukaemia and other cancers 细胞毒素的

radiotherapy /ˌreɪdɪəʊˈθerəpi/ *n*. the treatment of disease (especially cancer) by exposure to a radioactive substance 放射治疗

refractory /rɪˈfræktəri/ *adj*. (of a disease or medical condition) difficult to treat or cure

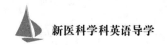

（疾病或体格状况）难以诊治的；难以治愈的

therapeutics /ˌθerəˈpjuːtɪks/ *n*. the branch of medicine concerned with the treatment of diseases 治疗学

metastasis /məˈtæstəsɪs/ *n*. the development of tumours in different parts of the body resulting from cancer that has started in another part of the body（瘤）转移

metastatic /ˌmetəˈstætɪk/ *adj*. relating to or affected by metastasis（癌细胞）转移性的；变形的；新陈代谢的

After reading

Task 11 **Build your vocabulary. Choose one word which can be used to replace the language shown in bold without changing the meaning of the sentence from the list below. Change forms and cases when necessary.**

comply with（*v.*） conclude（*v.*） equivalent（*adj.*） guarantee（*n.*） imply（*v.*）
methods（*n.*） obvious（*adj.*） presume（*v.*） proceed（*v.*） require（*v.*） specify（*v.*）
sum（*n.*）

1. If we can also **observe** GFP expressing in the sox7-/-doner chimera mice, it suggests that sox17 can be activated through other pathways in vivo, probably independent of Nodal signaling.

   _____

2. Mean SWE values decreased in testicles on the herniated side, but were not **equal** with those of contralateral testicles.

   _____

3. To compare advocates' and **state** leader's perspectives and understanding on the three main themes in children's mental health policies.

   _____

4. The belief that people **are morally obligated** toward fellow social group members, but not toward members of other groups, is an early-emerging feature of human cognition, arising out of domain-general processes in conceptual development.

   _____

5. This phenomenon has allowed genetic studies to be combined with biophysical measurements of single moving droplets, providing a **clear** view of motor protein control in vivo.

   _____

6. A new neuropsychological theory is proposed that accounts for many of these effects by **assuming** that positive affect is associated with increased brain dopamine levels.

   _____

7. To assess different **warranty** periods following a normal myocardial perfusion SPECT based on patients' clinical characteristics and the type of stress performed.

   _____

8. These **techniques** may have clinical value in objectively measuring change in a patient's shoulder posture as a result of a treatment program.　＿＿＿＿＿＿＿

9. There is ample evidence to **suggest** that posing leading questions is dangerous, in that it may elicit compliant responses that are not necessarily accurate.

　＿＿＿＿＿＿＿

10. The brain contains a significant **amount** of glycogen that is an order of magnitude smaller than that in muscle, but several-fold higher than the cerebral glucose content.　＿＿＿＿＿＿＿

Further reading

Koenig, I. R., Fuchs, O., Hansen, G., et al. (2017). What is Precision Medicine? *European Respiratory Journal*. 50(4).

McCann, S. R. (2022). Precision Medicine: Precision Viticulture. *Bone Marrow Transplant*. 57(5).

Mubarak, G., Zahir, F. R. (2022). Recent Major Transcriptomics and Epitranscriptomics Contributions toward Personalized and Precision Medicine. *Journal of Personalized Medicine*. 12(199).

Sisodiya, S. M. (2021). Precision Medicine and Therapies of the Future. *Epilepsia*. 62 (Suppl 2).

Solis, R. N., Silverman, D. A., Birkeland, A. C. (2022). Current Trends in Precision Medicine and Next-generation Sequencing in Head and Neck Cancer. *Current Treatment Options in Oncology*. 23(2).

Precision Medicine in Oncology

Guiding to learn

Precision cancer medicine (PCM) is an emerging paradigm in oncology, which includes tumour comprehensive genomic profiling (CGP) to enable molecularly guided therapy. However, cost-effectiveness analyses of PCM are faced with several challenges. Text A summarizes the improvements in the clinical management of patients with mCRC in the emerging era of precision medicine.

Discuss the following questions with your partners.

1. What challenges are the PCM now faced with?
2. What is precision cancer medicine?
3. What is the financial burden of PCM?

Task 1   Learn the following general academic vocabulary.

availability evidence financial identification significance variant appropriate evaluate potential relevant demonstrate framework initially insufficient register sequence adequately attribute emergence implementation mechanism obviously overall statistical alteration challenge entity evolve ratio assignment author interval utility comprehensive contrary definitive innovative paradigm accompany accumulate highlight prospective revolutionise scenario ongoing panel pose

Beginning to read

Task 2　Now read the text.

Text A

Cost-effectiveness of Precision Cancer Medicinecurrent Challenges in the Use of Next-Generation Sequencing for Comprehensive Tumour Genomic Proffling and the Role of Clinical Utility Framework

Konstantinos Christofyllakis et al

1. Precision cancer medicine（PCM）（精准癌症医学）is an emerging paradigm in cancer treatment striving to tailor anticancer therapy to the individual patient and treatment scenario. Originally，it referred to targeted or biomarker driven therapy. Examples of this approach include the use of monoclonal antibodies against cancers expressing a particular antigen/receptor，such as rituximab in CD20 positive Bcell lymphoma，or the use of tyrosine kinase inhibitors（TKIs）（酪氨酸激酶抑制剂）targeting a mutated kinase，such as EGFRTKIs in lung cancer with EGFR driver mutations. With increasing availability and evolution of hight rrough put technologies，such as next generation sequencing（NGS），the concept of PCM has evolved to include comprehensive genetic profiling（CGP）（综合遗传图谱）of individual tumours，in order to identify and target alterations that are patient and tumourspecific. This promise of personalized cancer therapy initially appeared alluring；however，the results of prospective trials have been sobering. The increased costs of comprehensive molecular tumour profiling for each individual patient and the cost of targeted therapy itself，pose the question of the costeffectiveness of this paradigm. Contrary to the broad application of PCM，streamlining its use in clinical scenarios where it is deemed to be clinically meaningful based on internationally recognised clinical frameworks can be an essential step in increasing its cost-effectiveness（成本效益）.

Clinical outcomes

2. The PCM approach has been tested in several prospective trials to date. The SHIVA trial randomized patients to receive either molecularly guided therapy or the physician's choice. Progression-free survival（PFS）was similar in both arms. Trédan et al reported one of the largest series to date，including 2,579 patients with advanced cancers in the ProfiLER trial. Molecularly guided treatment could be recommended for

27% of the patients, but only 6% received targeted therapy, achieving an overall response rate (ORR)(总体响应率)of 0.9%. The MOSCATO trial was a singlearm, prospective trial of highthroughput genomicsbased targeted therapy in patients with advanced cancers, reporting an ORR of 11%. In 33% of the patients (63/193), the PFS was at least 30% longer compared with previousline therapy (PFS2/PFS1 ratio > 1.3). This ratio is an emerging treatment endpoint in PCM, which calculates an intrapatient PFS ratio, by dividing the PFS interval associated with molecularly guided therapy (PFS2) by the PFS interval associated with the last prior systemic therapy (PFS1)(术前系统治疗). The WINTHER trial demonstrated a PFS2/PFS1 ratio of >1.5 in 22.4% of the patients. These modest outcomes may be attributed to intratumour heterogeneity, clonal evolution and emergence of resistance mechanisms under treatment with targeted agents. One important challenge that has been highlighted is to provide meaningful measures of outcome in smalln basket/umbrella trials. Innovative endpoints, like the PFS2/PFS1 ratio, used in the WINTHER and MOSCATO trials show promise in addressing this issue. These aforementioned trials represent "unguided", broad application of CGP in solid tumours. PCM has however revolutionised treatment in specific tumour entities, including nonsmall cell lung cancer (NSCLC)(非小细胞肺癌). Furthermore, in other entities, where molecularly guided treatment is not currently international standard, such as pancreatic cancer(胰腺癌), performing CGP with NGS achieved a relevant increase in overall survival among patients in whom an actionable molecular alteration was identified in a retrospective register analysis(回顾性注册分析). Within the MOSCATO trial itself, in the subgroup of patients with advanced biliary tract cancer(晚期胆道癌), treatment with molecularly guided therapy was associated with a lower risk for death, with an ORR of 33% and a PFS2/PFS1 ratio of >1.3 in 50% of the patients. Therefore, it is essential to correctly identify the tumour entities/clinical settings where PCM can lead to clinically meaningful improvements in outcome.

Costs

3. The sequencing of the first human genome in 2003 has been estimated to be between $500 million and $1 billion. The ongoing technological advancement in NGS techniques has led to a cost decrease of at least 5 orders of magnitude, and was projected in 2016 to lay < $1,000 per genome in 2020. A metaanalysis of trials conducted between 2005 and 2016 by Schwarze et al showed that cost estimates ranged from $555 to $5,169 for whole exome sequencing (WES)(全外显子组测序)and from $1,906 to $24,810 for whole genome sequencing (WGS)(全基因组测序). In one of the most recent analyses in 2016, Van Nimwegen et al calculated a per sample cost of €1,669 for WGS, €792 for WES and €333 for targeted gene panels(靶基因组).

4. However, the financial burden of PCM is currently primarily driven by the cost of targeted treatment itself, rather than by diagnostic measures. Pagès et al calculated the CGP cost per patient within the MOSCATO trial in France at €2,396, which was found to be only 6% of the total treatment costs; the cost of targeted therapy per patient was €31,269. Characteristically, anticancer drugs (54%) and hospitalizations (住院治疗) (35%) primarily accounted for the financial burden. For patients treated with chemotherapy, treatment costs were only slightly lower at € 29,183, driven primarily by higher hospitalization costs (+ 27%), whereas targeted therapy was mostly administered in the ambulatory setting. In conclusion, while the costs of genetic testing are continuously declining, the costs of targeted therapy remain significant and are not expected to decrease. On the other hand, CGP not only enables prediction of response to treatment, but also resistance, thus preventing further application of unnecessary (and costly) therapies. Lastly, "unguided" treatment may also be equally financially burdensome due to the increased need for hospital admissions.

Cost-effectiveness

5. In a recent systematic literature review by Schwarze et al in 2018, which discussed the role of WES and WGS in genetic diseases, cancer and infectious pathogens (病原体), the authors concluded that available evidence is currently insufficient to draw a definitive conclusion on whether PCM is costeffective. When estimating costeffectiveness in broad NGS panels (targeted panels, WES or WGS) in the context of PCM, one is faced with specific challenges. The first concerns evaluating the efficacy of PCM itself. The established measure of efficacy in the era of evidencebased medicine, the placebocontrolled phase Ⅲ (安慰剂对照期Ⅲ) randomised trial, is nearly impossible to apply in the context of PCM. The number of patients included in various umbrella or basket trials in PCM is insufficient to reach significant levels of statistical power for traditional endpoints, such as overall survival or PFS. Thus, Moscow et al suggested that "…. the clinical implementation of PCM might involve a tradeoff between a different standard of evidence for the adoption of new therapies, as is the case in patients with orphan diseases, in exchange for higher levels of precision in the assignment of treatment….". New clinical trial designs and endpoints, like the PFS2/PFS1 ration in the MOSCATO and WINTHER trials, are required to better quantify treatment benefit. Furthermore, there may be additional challenges when addressing the cost-effectiveness of PCM, as identified by Phillips et al. One such challenge is the difficulty of setting an appropriate comparator for NGS, i.e., single vs. multiple gene testing vs. no genetic testing. A single NGS panel could be used cost-effectively instead of multiple analyses of single genes, for example in NSCLC. Moreover, broad NGS panels often result in multiple secondary findings, or variants of unknown significance. Tracking the various cost and outcome trajectories

that derive from the clinical significance each of these accidentally identified variants is almost impossible in a costeffectiveness analysis. For example，accidental identification of a germline（生殖细胞系）BRCA1/2 mutation could lead to risk-reducing mastectomy（乳房切除术），initially causing an increase in healthcare costs. However，over time，costs probably would be reduced due to decreased breast cancer incidence. This also highlights the challenge of defining the time frame in which costs and outcomes apply. Certain costs，such as data storage or the need for additional tests （germline or family members），are difficult to depict when accompanied by findings of unclear significance. On the other hand，secondary germline data acquired with NGS，including genetic polymorphisms（多态性）predicting altered pharmacokinetics （药物动力学），may become relevant in future medical situations，and the potential benefits of their knowledge cannot be adequately depicted at the time of NGS testing.

From Molecular and Clinical Oncology，2022，16（1）

New words and expressions

paradigm /ˈpærədaɪm/ *n.* a typical example or pattern of sth 范式；范例；典范；样式

scenario /səˈnɑːrɪəʊ/ *n.* a description of how things might happen in the future 脚本；方案；设想；预测

prospective /prəˈspektɪv/ *adj.* expected to do sth or to become sth 预期的；潜在的；有望的；可能的；即将发生的；行将来临的

survival /sərˈvaɪv(ə)l/ *n.* the state of continuing to live or exist，often despite difficulty or danger 生存；存活；幸存

interval /ˈɪntəv(ə)l/ *n.* a period of time between two events 间隔；（时间上的）间隙；间歇

innovative /ˈɪnəveɪtɪv/ *adj.* introducing or using new ideas，ways of doing sth，etc.创新的；引进新思想的；采用新方法的；革新的

ongoing /ˈɒnɡəʊɪŋ/ *adj.* continuing to exist or develop 持续存在的，仍在进行的，不断发展的

primarily /praɪˈmerəli/ *adv.* mainly 主要地；根本地

After reading

Task 3   Read Text A again and answer the following questions.

1. Why is the financial burden of PCM currently primarily driven by the cost of targeted treatment?

2. When estimating cost-effectiveness in broad NGS panels (targeted panels, WES or WGS) in the context of PCM, what challenges are we faced with?

Task 4   Check your vocabulary. Fill in the blanks with the correct form of the words from the following box, each word can be used only once.

> achieve (*v.*)   conceive (*v.*)   automatic (*adj.*)   ensue (*v.*)   creat (*v.*)
> equilibrium(*n.*)   mathematics (*n.*)   manipulate (*v.*)   innovative (*adj.*)
> stable(*adj.*)   period(*n.*)   precede(*v.*)   series(*n.*)   section(*n.*)   tradition(*n.*)

1. It is apparent that some concepts and terms can be thought of as chronically. There are several substituent strategies that _____ this effect.

2. It is just as easy to imagine that Tempus's watches are better than Hora's as it is to _____ of the reverse.

3. People are more likely to have an _____ response to this information.

4. Fusarium Keratitis may completely destroy an eye within a few weeks and malignant glaucoma can _____ .

5. The best way you can predict your future is to _____ it.

6. Eventually, the entire building will come into _____ with the outdoor temperature.

7. Herzig (2004) states that in _____ , women and minorities take longer to progress with their degrees, and reach graduate and professional levels far less frequently than men.

8. Examining the competitive effects and responses of various plant species to interactions with other species has particular relevance to ecologists or conservation biologists trying to _____ species composition.

9. Its glass carving is beautiful and _____ .

10. In contrast to the first strategy, where the alliances were _____ and long term, first order alliances in the second strategy are transient and constantly changing.

Task 5   Build your vocabulary. Read the sentences below, decide which word in each bracket is more suitable.

1. Hypoxia can (occur/takes) since oxygen will be limiting due to a lower partial pressure of oxygen outside of the plant.

2. These theories contend that children should not be seen as (inert/passive) receptors of adult instruction but as active agents who effectively negotiate with and evaluate their social world.

3. The crosses performed are outlined in the chart below. Additionally in preparation of the marker one and three backcross an initial cross of unknown virgin females and the (respective/single) maker males was performed.

4. It may be correct to then (infer/imply) that biological systems can arise more quickly by employing ND architectures than otherwise.

5. These researchers argue that because of the (accelerating/catching up) process of globalization, cultures are moving and mixing, thereby, resulting in a hybridization (Hermans et al., 1998) of cultures.

6. An analysis of the environmental and ecological conditions imposed on creatures during this time frame can help elucidate the (important/major) factors that drove terrestriality in tetrapods.

7. This theory, however, is still limited because reduced gene flow itself may not cause speciation; furthermore, it is only with an accumulation of many neutral or weakly under dominant rearrangements, linked to isolation loci, that a larger (piece/portion) of the genome can be affected.

8. Temperatures also (ebb and flow/fluctuate) on daily and seasonal scales, further adding to the variability in temperature-related impacts on processes such as N-mineralization.

9. Leptin may also (award/contribute) to hypertension through its effects on circulating white blood cells.

10. The (concentration/focus) of these studies includes drought, cold, heat, salinity, and hypoxia.

Guiding to learn

Task 6　Learn the following general academic vocabulary.

constitutive variability variant abnormal distinct feature regulation relevant corresponding initially rely sequence approximately emerging promoter subsequent summarize unpredictable alteration fundamental instability stable substitution transition whereas domain inhibition transformation utilization comprehensive comprise differentiation reverse accumulation conformation highlight induce predominant mediate trigger integrity

Beginning to read

Task 7　Now read the text.

Text B

Clinical Management of Metastatic Colorectal Cancer in the Era of Precision Medicine

Fortunato Ciardiello et al

1. Colorectal cancer（CRC）（结肠直肠癌）is the third most common cancer in males and the second most common in females, with approximately 1.9 million new cases and 0.9 million deaths in 2020 worldwide. CRC incidence has increased in recent years. It represents approximately 10% of all cancers and is the second most frequent cause of cancer deaths. Therefore, CRC is a global public health challenge in terms of morbidity, mortality, and utilization of health care services, including increasingly high medical costs.

2. Approximately 20% of patients with CRC have metastases at the time of diagnosis, whereas up to 50% of patients with initially localized disease will develop metastases. CRC can spread by lymphatic（淋巴的）and hematogenous（造血的）dissemination as well as by contiguous and peritoneal routes. The most frequent metastatic sites are regional lymph nodes, liver, lungs, and peritoneum（腹膜）. The prognosis of patients who have metastatic CRC（mCRC）has significantly improved in the past 20 years with the introduction of more effective therapeutic approaches, including surgery of liver and lung metastases and novel anticancer drugs. However, mCRC in most cases remains a noncurable disease（无法治愈的疾病）.

3. This review summarizes the improvement in the clinical management of patients with mCRC in the emerging era of precision medicine. An individual, personalized therapeutic approach based on comprehensive knowledge of the complex genetic and environmental bases of the disease is required to achieve long-term control of mCRC with significantly better quality and quantity of life.

Molecular Pathogenic Routes of Colorectal Cancer Development

4. CRC is a heterogenous disease characterized by a plethora of molecular alterations that determine the dysregulation of different signaling pathways, leading to tumor onset, progression, and invasiveness. The high intertumor and intratumor

variability at different genetic levels highlights the complex molecular biology of the neoplasm, which, in turn, affects tumor response to therapies and patient survival. 8 Even in the presence of a recognized and druggable gene alteration, the antitumor activity of the corresponding matched target therapy remains unpredictable. Hence, better knowledge of the multiple developmental trajectories of CRC is fundamental to identify and tackle cancer vulnerabilities and to change the clinical course of the disease.

5. Molecular heterogeneity may already be found at premalignant stages. This is determined by genetic and epigenetic regulations, which will influence different CRC molecular profiles. In this regard, 3 distinct pathways have been identified in the pathogenesis of CRC: chromosomal instability, high microsatellite instability (MSI-H) (微卫星高度不稳定性), and CpG island methylator phenotype (CIMP) (CpG 岛甲基化表型).

6. Chromosomal instability (染色体不稳定性)is reported in approximately 65% to 70% of sporadic CRC and refers to an abnormal accumulation of gain or loss of entire regions of chromosomes that, in turn, results in chromosome number alterations, chromosome amplifications, and/or loss of heterozygosity (LOH) (杂合性丢失). In 1990, Fearon and Volgestein described a multistep genetic model for the adenoma-to-carcinoma sequence that represented a milestone in the understanding of CRC initiation and progression. The first step in the tumorigenic (致瘤的) process is silencing, mutation, or LOH of the gatekeeper adenomatous polyposis coli (APC) gene. Loss of APC function causes the constitutive activation of WNT signaling, which controls the proliferation, differentiation, and renewal of intestinal stem cells, leading to the transformation of normal epithelium to early adenoma. A subsequent accumulation of gene alterations, including KRAS, TP53, and LOH 18q, occurs during the transition from adenoma to carcinoma. Finally, dysregulation of the phosphoinositide–3 kinase (PI3K) and transforming growth factor β (TGF-β) (转化生长因子 β)pathways is frequently observed in later stages.

7. The second group of CRCs (approximately 15%—20%) is characterized by a deficit in the DNA mismatch-repair (dMMR) system, leading to an abnormal accumulation of gene mutations. The integrity of the dMMR machinery (MLH1, MSH2, MSH6, and PMS2 proteins) is necessary for recognizing, correcting, and thus preventing errors during DNA replication. A dysfunctional dMMR system causes the generation of novel microsatellite fragments and of neoantigens, thus determining the MSI-H phenotype. Germline mutations in one of the dMMR genes are the hallmark of hereditary nonpolyposis CRC or Lynch syndrome, in which there is an increased risk of developing different gastrointestinal malignancies, including CRC.

8. The serrated neoplasia pathway (锯齿状肿瘤形成路径) is the third pathogenic (致病的) route in CRC development. Epigenomic instability of serrated neoplasia

relies on the dysregulation of CpG island methylation. Aberrant hypermethylation in the promoter region of suppressor genes results in gene silencing and favors tumor onset (CIMP phenotype). Of note, nonhereditary, sporadic MSI-H tumors also could be the result of MLH1 silencing and are strictly associated with BRAF valine-to-glutamate substitution at codon 600 (V600E) mutations. Epigenetic silencing of other tumor suppressor genes, such as MGMT, p16INK4, and IGFBP7, could play a significant role in the development of CIMP CRC. However, a subgroup of MSI-H tumors could also present features of serrated neoplasia.

Mutational Landscape of Metastatic Colorectal Cancer

9. Major efforts have been made to better understand the genomic landscape of CRC and to identify druggable (可靶向的) mutations, with the aim of developing a truly precision medicine-based, personalized treatment for each patient. The effective development of precision oncology for patients with mCRC has been more challenging than expected. This may be explained in part by the genetic heterogeneity of these tumors, the paucity of druggable targets, and the complex interplay between different signaling pathways that could allow cancer cells to escape single-target inhibition.

10. After more than 20 years of translational and clinical investigation, targeting the epidermal growth factor receptor (EGFR) (表皮生长因子受体) family and its intracellular signaling pathways still represents the most relevant keystone for the targeted molecular treatment of mCRC.

From CA Cancer J Clin，2022，72(4)

After reading

Task 8　Build your vocabulary.

Directions: Match the following words with their corresponding definitions and Chinese equivalents.

English: integrity　trigger (*v.*)　predominant　heterogenous　epigenetic　alteration approximately　abnormal　instability　variability　dysfunctional

Chinese: 完整性　触发　不正常的　改变　卓越的　大概　不稳定　易变性　异种的 功能障碍的　后成的

Paras. 1—7

	English	Chinese	Definition
1.	_____	_____	a. having superior power and influence
2.	_____	_____	b. the quality of a situation in which things are likely to change or fail suddenly
3.	_____	_____	c. the quality of being honest and having strong moral principles
4.	_____	_____	d. put in motion or move to act
5.	_____	_____	e. the quality of being subject to variation
6.	_____	_____	f. a change to sth that makes it different
7.	_____	_____	g. used to show that sth is almost, but not completely, accurate or correct
8.	_____	_____	h. different from what is usual or expected, especially in a way that is worrying, harmful or not wanted
9.	_____	_____	i. not originating within the body; of foreign origin
10.	_____	_____	j. not working normally or properly
11.	_____	_____	k. of or relating to epigenesis

Guiding to learn

Task 9 Learn the following general academic vocabulary from the word bank.

metabolism optimize density diffusion transmit dynamic processes integrity crucial metabolic consume generating normal accumulation fulfill alterations deactivation systemic challenging emerged transfer contrast maintain fundamental

Beginning to read

Task 10   Now read the text.

Text C

Targeting Mitochondrial Metabolism for
Precision Medicine in Cancer
Lourdes Sainero-Alcolado et al

Introduction: Tumor metabolism

1. Cancer cells are characterized by the ability to proliferate uncontrollably in contrast to normal cells, which are tightly regulated. To maintain rapid cell proliferation(快速细胞增殖), tumor cells activate and/or modify metabolic pathways to obtain more energy, known as metabolic reprogramming. This research field has gained special interest during the latest decade due to new insights into its fundamental importance and the development of novel biochemical and molecular tools. In 2011, Douglas Hanahan and Robert A. Weinberg included metabolic reprogramming as one of the capabilities acquired during malignant transformation, i. e., one of the hallmarks of cancer.

2. In the 1920s, Otto Warburg described that tumor cells consume high amounts of glucose to produce lactate via "aerobic glycolysis"（有氧糖酵解）regardless of the presence of oxygen, generating only two molecules of ATP per molecule of glucose, versus the 36 ATP molecules produced during oxidative phosphorylation（OXPHOS）（氧化磷酸化）in normal cells. To overcome the 18-fold difference in efficiency, glycolysis is activated by upregulation of glucose transporters（including GLUT1）to increase glucose uptake and by overexpression of the rate-limiting enzyme in glycolysis, hexokinase‑2, and lactate dehydrogenase（LDHA）（乳酸脱氢酶）. The increase in glycolytic flux results in accumulation of glycolytic intermediates that supply different biosynthetic pathways to fulfill the demands of proliferation, e.g. the pentose phosphate pathway（PPP）for production of ribose and cytosolic nicotinamide adenine dinucleotide phosphate（NADPH）（还原型烟酰胺腺嘌呤二核苷酸磷酸）used for nucleotide synthesis and antioxidants; as well as one carbon metabolism（碳代谢）necessary for mitochondrial NADPH production, methylation, and nucleotide synthesis.

3. The metabolic alterations in tumor cells are mainly driven by aberrant activation of the phosphatidylinositol－3 kinase-protein kinase B-mammalian target of rapamycin（PI3K-AKT-mTOR）pathway and activation of oncogenes such as MYC, RAS, and hypoxia-inducible factor 1（HIF－1）（缺氧诱导因子）, as well as mutations or deactivation of tumor suppressor genes including p53 and PTEN.

The Warburg effect and the relevance of OXPHOS

4. Warburg hypothesized in 1956 that tumor cells rely more on aerobic glycolysis due to an injury in respiration, which led to the misconception that cancer cells have a defective oxidative metabolism（氧化代谢缺陷）. However, Warburg's experiments indicated that tumors consume oxygen at a lower rate compared to their increased glucose consumption. Several studies have demonstrated that many cancer cells have the capacity to oxidize glucose via OXPHOS in their fully functional mitochondria. Moreover, inhibition of glycolysis does not prevent tumorigenesis. For instance, inhibition of the pyruvate kinase M2 isoform, responsible for the last step of glycolysis, still results in tumor formation in a breast cancer model. Furthermore, inhibiting LDHA increases mitochondrial respiration in mammary tumor cells, proving that oxidative metabolism still is functional. Therefore, cancer cells may depend equally or predominantly on OXPHOS for ATP supply, with the exemption of tumors with mutations in the tricarboxylic acid（TCA）（三羧酸）cycle enzyme genes SDH, IDH, and FH, important during mitochondrial respiration. However, tumors carrying such mutations are still dependent on mitochondrial activity, and are remodeling their metabolism to optimize production of reactive oxygen species（ROS）（活性氧簇）and produce TCA cycle intermediates necessary for cell proliferation.

Mitochondria

5. Mitochondria are the organelles responsible for energy production in cells. The discovery of the mitochondrial genome（线粒性基因组）（mtDNA）and phylogenetic gene analysis showed that mitochondria are descendants of an endosymbiotic α-proteobacteria. They consist of an outer（OMM）and an inner membrane（IMM）（内膜）, limiting the intermembrane mitochondrial space, and an electron-dense matrix. The IMM folds in the matrix forming the cristae, which contain the mitochondria respiratory machinery and whose density varies depending on the energy demand. The OMM is permeable, allowing diffusion of molecules up to kDalton via the porin voltage dependent anion channel, receiving signals that will be transmitted into mitochondria. It also serves as a contact site for interaction with other organelles including the endoplasmic reticulum（内质网）, lysosomes, peroxisomes, endosomes, the plasma membrane, and lipid droplets.

6. Mitochondria are highly dynamic and stay in constant turnover through

mitogenesis，mitophagy，and fusion-fission processes. They control a vast number of cellular processes related to metabolism，apoptosis，redox homeostasis（氧化还原稳态），calcium signaling，and iron metabolism，thus their integrity is fundamental for the cell.

From Cell Death Differ，2022，29（7）

New words and expressions

intelligence /ɪnˈtelɪdʒəns/ *n*. the ability to learn，understand and think in a logical way about things；the ability to do this well 智力；才智；智慧

device /dɪˈvaɪs/ *n*. an object or a piece of equipment that has been designed to do a particular job 装置；仪器；器具；设备

intervention /ˌɪntəˈvenʃən/ *n*. the act of intervening in a situation 干涉；干预

predominantly /prɪˈdɒmɪnəntli/ *adv*. mostly，mainly 主要地；多数情况下

automatically /ˌɒtəˈmætɪkli/ *adv*. in a reflex manner 自动地；机械地

qualitative /ˈkwɒlɪtətɪv/ *adj*. connected with how good sth is，rather than with how much of it there is 质量的；定性的；性质的

protocol /ˈprəʊtəkɒl/ *n*. a plan for performing a scientific experiment or medical treatment 科学实验计划；医疗方案

expertise /ˌekspɜːˈtiːz/ *n*. expert knowledge or skill in a particular subject，activity or job 专业知识；专长；专门知识；专门技能

manually /ˈmænjʊəli/ *adv*. using your hands or your physical strength rather than your mind 用手地；手动地；人工地

potential /pəˈtenʃ(ə)l/ *adj*. that can develop into sth or be developed in the future 潜在的；可能的

specificity /ˌspesɪˈfɪsəti/ *n*. the quality of being specific 明确性；具体性；独特性

primary /ˈpraɪməri/ *adj*. main；most important 主要的；最重要的；基本的

After reading

Task 11　Build your vocabulary. Choose one word which can be used to replace the language shown in bold without changing the meaning of the sentence from the list below. Change forms and cases when necessary.

affect(*v*.)　capillary(*n*.)　notion(*n*.)　decade(*n*.)　emphasise(*v*.)　expose(*v*.)
generate(*v*.)　consequent(*adj*.)　pertinent(*adj*.)　predict(*v*.)　select(*v*.)
signify(*v*.)　structure(*n*.)　undergo(*v*.)

1. Over the relatively short time of **ten years**, actual life-table survival probabilities decline approximately linearly. _____

2. We will revise the contents of Social Studies, Civics and Moral Education, and History, to **stress** nation-building. _____

3. Cracking can **uncover** rebar which makes the rebar more vulnerable to corrosion.

   _____

4. The sum of these modifications occurring during the Devonian and Carboniferous led to the eventual filling of the terrestrial realm with vertebrate life, forever altering the **organisation** and ecology of terrestrial communities. _____

5. The replacement names **indicated** the arrival of settlers, who became the focal point of an area, and this ignorance to the attributes of the land represented a small step toward uniformity. _____

6. These developing forests **created** oxygen as a photosynthetic waste product, thus increasing its abundance in the atmosphere and making the land a much more suitable place for animal life. _____

7. Sustained periods of rain further dilute the pathogen in aquatic reservoirs and epidemics occur during the rainy season, presumably through immigration of infected individuals and the **result** secondary route of transmission.

   _____

8. Other complications of angiogenesis occur primarily because arterial walls are normally free of microvessels except in the atherosclerotic plaques where there are dense networks of **small blood vessels** known as the vasa vasorum.

   _____

9. It appears as if his **concept** is based solely on his own similarity judgment. Without a phylogenetic diagnosis, we lack a measure for selecting between alternative mechanisms for explaining this disjunct distribution. _____

10. I will grow seedlings at the normal Earth pressure of 101 kPa. Past data has already shown that low atmospheric pressures do not negatively **effect** plant growth from a visual standpoint. _____

Further reading

Christofyllakis, K., Bittenbring, J. T., Thurner, L., et al.(2022). Cost-effectiveness of Precision Cancer Medicine—Current Challenges in the Use of Next Generation Sequencing for Comprehensive Tumour Genomic Profiling and the Role of Clinical Utility Frameworks (Review). *Molecular and Clinical Oncology*. 16(1).

Ciardiello, F., Ciardiello, D., Martini, G., et al. (2022). Clinical Management of Metastatic Colorectal Cancer in the Era of Precision Medicine. *CA Cancer J Clin*. 72(4).

Hu, M., Wang, Z., Wu, Z., et al. (2022). Circulating Tumor Cells in Colorectal Cancer in the Era of Precision Medicine. *Journal of Molecular Medicine*（*Berlin*）. 100(2).

Middleton，G.，Robbins，H.，Andre，F.，et al. (2022). A State-of-the-art Review of Stratified Medicine in Cancer: Towards a Future Precision Medicine Strategy in Cancer. *Annals of Oncology*. 33(2).

Sainero-Alcolado，L.，Liaño-Pons，J.，Ruiz-Pérez，M. V.，et al. (2022). Targeting Mitochondrial Metabolism for Precision Medicine in Cancer. *Cell Death Differ*. 29(7).

Unit 3
Genomics in Precision Medicine

Guiding to learn

The completion of the Human Genome Project（HGP）in 2001 opened the floodgates to a deeper understanding of medicine. The new precision medicine，where genome sequencing and data analysis are essential components，allows tailored diagnosis and treatment according to the information from the patients' own genome and specific environmental factors. Biliary tract cancers are a group of heterogeneous and rare malignancies that arise from any point of the biliary tract and are uniformly associated with poor prognosis. A "pathway" driven approach targeting the cumulative influence of psycho-social，epigenetic，or cellular factors is likely to be more effective.

Discuss the following questions with your partners.

1. What are the public and private cloud computing platforms disadvantages?
2. What can biliary tract cancers be subdivided into?
3. How can the researchers optimize the therapeutic potential of precision medicine?

Task 1　Learn the following general academic vocabulary.

analyze assumption distribution interpret principle variation complex computation feature impact institute maintain normalization participant relevant component consent considerable constant core dominant initially maximum sequence approximately goal mechanism parallel status subsequently generate oriente transition precede underlying dynamic intervention submission manipulation medium scenario assembly conceive enormous

Beginning to read

Task 2 Now read the text.

Text A

Human Genomics Projects and Precision Medicine
F. Carrasco Ramiro et al

1. The completion of the Human Genome Project (HGP)（人类基因组计划）has been compared to the first human moon landing. Both massive projects involved the effort of many scientists, collaboration of many countries and massive technological development. Nowadays we are unable to conceive science without technology, which has made a significant impact in genomics as it is currently possible to sequence not one but thousands of human genomes per year around the world and this amount keeps increasing. Many companies are improving and developing new sequencing technologies, raising concern among institutions and companies regarding the storage and analysis of the generated data.

2. The knowledge generated through the HGPs has changed genomics and is entering clinical practice. Genome sequencing and data analysis are essential components of the new precision (personalized) medicine, delivering customized diagnosis and treatment. In addition, crucial for this new kind of medicine are the knowledge of underlying mechanisms of diseases, the understanding of environment-biology interactions, and evidence-based interventions. Using all this information it should be possible to plot the transition from health to disease of an individual. Pharmacogenomics, the combination of pharmacology and genomics, plays a crucial role. Clinicians could advise people on lifestyle changes when treatments might not be necessary, or even to consider preventive measures when there is a high likelihood of developing disease. The new P4 (predictive, preventive, precise and participatory) medicine will require new standards and policies for handling biological and health care information about individuals. Genomes may contain information that people wish to keep confidential, and predictions of future health status raise complex questions about how much people want to know or want others to know. Complex data sets need to be handled securely and interpreted knowledgeably and thoroughly.

3. After the Human Genome Project (HGP) was completed, the genome sequencing（基因组测序）field started to work in a completely different way, mainly

since 2005 when the Next-Generation Sequencing（NGS）era began. In this scenario, Roche played an instrumental role acquiring the 454 technology and launching its Genome Sequencer instrument. Soon, the first Solexa sequencer, the Genome Analyzer, appeared, and shortly after the company was acquired by Illumina. This fast development of the NGS technology brought considerable challenges to these companies, and after a few years of struggle the Illumina technology consolidated its current dominant position, and Roche discontinued its platform in 2016.

NGS technologies

4. Several companies currently offer different technologies that serve one or several niche applications, all sharing two common features. First, the nucleic acid molecules within the sample must be prepared in order to be sequenced. This always involves a ligation step with universal adapters to their 5′ and 3′ ends, that in some technologies is preceded by the fragmentation and end repairing of the nucleic acid molecules. Also, in some of the technologies, a clonal amplification of the molecules after the adapter ligation is required. Second, thousands to billions of molecules from this 'library' are sequenced in parallel, generating a massive amount of sequences that is many orders of magnitude above what a Sanger sequencer can deliver. For a detailed revision of NGS technologies see Goodwin *et al*. A summary of some of them is presented below.

5. Illumina's core technology is based on clonal solid-state bridge amplification of DNA or cDNA molecules that are subsequently sequenced by synthesis with a DNA polymerase and fluorescently labeled, reversibly blocked deoxy nucleotide triphosphates（dNTPs）（脱氧核苷酸三磷酸）. The result is an enormous throughput per run and the lowest cost per sequenced Gbase on the market, which makes Illumina the platform of choice for most NGS applications. Illumina has also developed a wide range of instruments that differ in the maximum read length that can be obtained（100—300 bp）as well as in the number of reads per run（14 million—10 billion）and this allows each laboratory to choose the instrument that suits its needs best. In 2014 Illumina launched the HiSeq X instrument, which can sequence a human genome at 30x coverage, or greater, for less than $1000 including consumables, wet-lab labor, instrument depreciation, and basic data analysis. After the recent introduction in January 2017 of the NovaSeq series, the productivity will benefit from faster runs and the cost might be reduced in 2018 with the arrival of a new type of flow cell.

6. Thermo Fisher Scientific is present in the NGS market with two different technologies: SOLiD6 and Ion Torrent. SOLiD features short read lengths and long run times with the advantage of checking every nucleotide position（核苷酸位置）twice. Ion Torrent is based on standard chemistry and semiconductor technology, succeeding in the disease-specific amplicon sequencing field due to the ease of use and the fast run

times, which match quite well the typical needs in a clinical environment.

7. Among the single-molecule and long-read technologies, Pacific Biosciences (PacBio) instruments can provide average read lengths within the 10—18 kb range, based on the single-molecule real-time (SMRT) sequencing technology(单分子实时测序技术). It is the technology of choice for de novo assembly of genomes, studying long-range structural variations or even full length transcript sequencing. Its limited throughput increases significantly the cost per sequenced gigabase. However, although it cannot be used routinely for human genome resequencing, it is currently being used to improve the quality of the reference human genomes in different projects. PacBio has recently claimed a roadmap including a 30x increase of productivity by the end of 2018 which would allow denovo sequencing of a human genome for $1000 in reagents.

8. Oxford Nanopore Technologies (ONT) is playing a significant role in the long-read world, with its miniaturized nanopore-based MinION sequencer that could suit on-site clinical sequencing applications. The technology is in constant development and can provide reads of several kilobases in length. The company has also started an early-access program to its PromethION platform, a high productivity instrument based on the same nanopore technology that is intended to compete with Illumina's HiSeq X. ONT is also launching a medium-throughput instrument called GridIONX5.

9. Another interesting approach to long-read technologies is the use of chemically barcoded short-length reads to informatically rebuild synthetic long reads which can be more informative, trying to get the best of both worlds. Among this group there are companies such as Illumina, 10xGenomics and iGenomeX.

10. As noted, this is a highly dynamic field and, currently, there are several technologies in different stages of development that could step in the NGS world in the near future: Genapsys (electronics based), Genia (nanopore), Illumina Firefly (semiconductor), Nanostring (enzyme-free hybridization), GnuBio (FRET-based) and Electron Optica (electron microscopy).

11. Data management, protection and security: public repositories Data management in genomics has been considered as a "four headed beast" due to the computational challenges that are faced across the lifecycle of a data set: acquisition, storage, distribution and analysis. Only in terms of data acquisition and storage, in 2025 the projected computational needs are calculated to be about 1 zetta-bases per year and 2—40 exa-bytes per year, respectively, as the total amount of sequence data doubles approximately every seven months.

12. Regarding the protection of data distribution and analysis, homomorphic encryption systems(同态加密系统), which allow manipulation and analysis for certain controlled queries without publishing raw data, seem to be the path to follow in future research, but nowadays they are too demanding in terms of computing needs.

13. The storage of the huge amount of data produced by sequencing technologies,

into public and private clouds raises concerns about privacy and security. Initially, human genome projects were based on the principles of open access, requiring the sequences to be deposited in public repositories, assuming that there was no risk of identification of participants or donors. This assumption was overturned after realizing that data from individuals could be distinguished in Genome Wide Association Studies (GWAS)(全基因组关联研究) just using summary statistics. Newer projects try to address this issue requiring managed access to data consented for biomedical research.

From Gene Therapy, 2017, 24(9)

New words and expressions

genomics /dʒɪˈnɒmɪks/ *n*. the study of genomes 基因组学

precision /prɪˈsɪʒ(ə)n/ *n*. the quality of being exact, accurate and careful 精确;准确;细致

pharmacology /fɑːməˈkɒlədʒi/ *n*. the scientific study of drugs and their use in medicine 药物学;药理学

participatory /pɑːˌtɪsɪˈpeɪtəri/ *adj*. a participatory system, activity, or role involves a particular person or group of people taking part in it (体制、活动、角色)参与式的

confidential /ˌkɒnfɪˈdenʃ(ə)l/ *adj*. meant to be kept secret and not told to or shared with other people 机密的;保密的;秘密的

amplification /æmplɪfɪˈkeɪʃn/ *n*. the amount of increase in signal power or voltage or current expressed as the ratio of output to input 扩大(充);膨胀

sequence /ˈsiːkwəns/ *v*. to identify the order in which a set of genes or parts of molecules are arranged 测定(整套基因或分子成分的)序列

semiconductor /ˌsemɪkənˈdʌktə(r)/ *n*. a solid substance that conducts electricity in particular conditions, better than insulators but not as well as conductors 半导体

miniaturize /ˈmɪnətʃəraɪz/ *vt*. to make a much smaller version of sth 使微型化;使成为缩影

molecule /ˈmɒlɪkjuːl/ *n*. the smallest unit, consisting of a group of atoms, into which a substance can be divided without a change in its chemical nature 分子

repository /rɪˈpɒzətri/ *n*. a place where sth is stored in large quantities 仓库;贮藏室;存放处

manipulation /məˌnɪpjʊˈleɪʃən/ *n*. the action of touching with the hands (or the skillful use of the hands) or by the use of mechanical means 操纵;操作法

deposit /dɪˈpɒzɪt/ *vt*. to leave a layer of sth on the surface of sth, especially gradually and over a period of time 使沉积;使沉淀;使淤积

dissemination /dɪˌsemɪˈneɪʃən/ *n*. the property of being diffused or dispersed 散播

implementation /ˌɪmplɪmenˈteɪʃən/ *n*. the act of accomplishing some aim or executing some order 贯彻;生效;完成

After reading

Task 3　Read Text A again and answer the following questions.

1. What's the significance of the completion of the Human Genome Project (HGP)?
2. What's the basis of Illumina's core technology?
3. What's the function of data management in genomics?

Task 4　Check your vocabulary. Fill in the blanks with the correct form of the words from the following box, each word can be used only once.

coordinate(*v.*)	discrete (*adj.*)	estimate (*n.*)	geography (*n.*)	norm (*n.*)
pole(*n.*)	preposition(*n.*)	rational(*adj.*)	scheme(*n.*)	source(*n.*)　task(*n.*)
underline(*v.*)				

1. It is not possible to disentangle the effects of the different intervention elements like social _____ feedback, a high-profile messenger, and behavioral instruction.

2. The variable year was treated as a _____ variable to determine differences between different years for opioid prescribing.

3. The networks of the brainstem and spinal cord that _____ locomotion and body orientation in lamprey are described.

4. Hospital characteristics included bed size, teaching status, _____, staffing ratios, surgical volume, and frequency of each procedure type.

5. Rigid endoscopes with effective light _____ enable the relatively narrow middle ear cavity to be viewed clearly, in detail, and completely, allowing surgeons to work effectively in the area.

6. English input and output accounted for most of the variance in English _____ score.

7. To balance patient characteristics between the 2 groups, we used PS _____ to derive individual weights.

8. In conclusion, inequalities in health and pain are determined by a number of variables and differences in lifetime exposure to various factors, and the pattern noted between acute and chronic pain with respect to SEP necessitates tracking pain from the acute stages in order to identify the _____ elements that affect pain management and treatment within the socio-economic strata.

9. Because both options have the same expected value, a _____ individual would see these options as equivalent and have no driven preference between the two options.

10. Is a multi-sport type of helmet appropriate and safe for use in _____ vaulting?

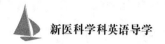

Task 5 Build your vocabulary. Read the sentences below, decide which word in each bracket is more suitable.

1. This test presents an ability to distinguish（deficient/inadequate）from normal males with 100% negative predictive value（NPV）at 30%（of normal G6PD activity）cut-off.

2. While the PCA（tale/plot）suggests that NSOI can resemble sarcoidosisxA1xAF TED or NSOIxA1xAF we remain uncertain as to whether some NSOI is representative of a fourth disease distinct from the other three.

3. Another critical（transition/transit）point，for high-risk patients，is from surgery to chemotherapy.

4. Because of its chemical properties，we expected that this compound would be （correct/appropriate）for stable liposomal loading while providing suitable MR imaging properties for application in image-guided drug delivery.

5. Exclusion Rights—the right to determine who may use the resource. An actor with rights up to level 3 is considered a（proprietor/landlord）.

6. This study explores how IM subspecialty professional（communes/societies）support their clinician-educator members.

7. A small writing group was（convened/gathered）to complete the guidelines manuscript.

8. The United States relies on space more than any other nation. American life is informed and connected by a vast network of hundreds of（stations/satellites）silently in orbit overhead.

9. Another critical（topic/issue）is how mothers with suspected or confirmed Ebola virus disease will safely feed their infants in these settings.

10. The study did not otherwise（deviate/divert）from the original protocol.

Guiding to learn

Task 6 Learn the following general academic vocabulary.

available constitutive significantly vary administration commission normally strategy demonstrate initially approximately confer option overall statistical subsequently alteration capacity expansion modification transition assigne domain enhance inhibition reveal transformation eventually highlight schedule uniformly duration preliminary trigger ongoing

Beginning to read

Task 7   Now read the text.

Text B

Precision Medicine Targeting FGFR2 Genomic Alterations in Advanced Cholangiocarcinoma: Current State and Future Perspectives

Miguel Zugman et al

1. Biliary tract cancers (BTCs)(胆道癌) are a group of heterogenous and rare malignancies that arise from any point of the biliary tract yet are uniformly associated with poor prognosis. BTCs are subdivided in intrahepatic cholangiocarcinoma (ICCA)(肝内胆管细胞癌), extrahepatic cholangiocarcinoma (ECCA)(肝外胆管癌) and gallbladder cancer(胆囊癌). ICCA originates from within the liver parenchyma, whereas ECCA can arise from any portion of the biliary tract outside of the liver, which can be further classified as hilar or distal cholangiocarcinoma. Incidence worldwide is increasing, both from ICCA and ECCA. The estimated number of new cases of primary liver cancer, including hepatocellular carcinoma and biliary cancers (肝细胞癌和胆道癌), to have occurred globally in 2020, were of 906.000, of which ICCA accounts for approximately 10%—15%.

2. The therapy of choice for advanced BTCs was established by the ABC - 02 phase III trial, OS was significantly improved with gemcitabine and cisplatin versus gemcitabine. A phase Ⅱ, non-randomized, single-arm clinical trial investigated the addition of nab-paclitaxel to gemcitabine-cisplatin. Median PFS was 12.2 months, and median OS was 19.2 months, which compares favorably to historical controls. Lately, positive results with the addition of durvalumab to chemotherapy was achieved in the TOPAZ - 1 trial. In the study, durvalumab combined with cisplatin and gemcitabine conferred a 20% reduction in the risk of death compared with gemcitabine and cisplatin alone, meeting the primary endpoint of the trial, PFS and response rate were also improved with the combination. Although FOLFIRINOX is an effective regimen in pancreatic cancer, in advanced biliary cancers it was not superior to gemcitabine and cisplatin in the phase Ⅱ randomized trial PRODIGE 38 AMEBICA. For second-line chemotherapy, results are less encouraging. Randomized trials identified mFOLFOX or 5FU plus liposomal irinotecan as regimens considered second-line options with improvements in OS for patients who have progressed after gemcitabine-

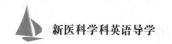

based treatment，although more efficacious treatments are in need.

3. Biomarkers are present in varying patterns among ICCA and ECCA，and such differences highlight tumor-specific oncogenic pathways. Some of these biomarkers predicted the response to fibroblast growth factor receptor（FGFR）（成纤维细胞生长因子受体）inhibitors，which target FGFR2-fusions in ICCA. The FGFR2 belongs to the FGFR family of tyrosine kinases receptors. The family consists of 4 genes that encode single-pass transmembrane receptors that bind to FGF on the extracellular domain. Ligand binding trigger a signaling cascade that may exercise several cellular functions，including cell survival. It is estimated that FGFR2 genomic alterations are present in around 10—15% of ICCA，most of them consisting of fusions，but also different aberrations can drive oncogenic transformation，such as mutations and amplifications，which may account for up to 3% of the cases.

4. Chromosomal rearrangements cause intragenic translocations that encode functional proteins derived from each of the original proteins. FGFR2 partners up with other proteins with strong dimerization capacity，resulting in constitutive receptor activation and downstream signaling. Normally，FGF-FGFR signaling is triggered by the ligand-dependent receptor dimerization. The activation of the receptor leads to intracellular phosphorylation of receptor kinase domains，a cascade of intracellular signaling，and gene transcription. FGFR2 constitutive kinase activity is linked to oncogene addictive pathways including the RAS-MAPK，JAK-STAT，and PIK3-AKT-mTOR，promoting progressive growth，invasiveness，epithelial-mesenchymal transition（上皮-间质转化）and neo angiogenesis（血管生成），Single point mutations have been shown as well to increase FGFR activity by enhancing ligand binding of altering ligand specificity，they can also impair autoinhibitory brakes，which eventually turn to constitutive activity of the receptor kinase domain. All this alterations in FGFR genes，including activating mutations，chromosomal translocations，gene fusions，and gene amplifications，can result in ligand-independent signaling which increase receptor kinase activity.

5. Pemigatinib is a tyrosine multi-kinase inhibitor that blocks FGFR1－3，with weaker activity against FGFR4. It has been shown that pemigatinib inhibits the growth of tumor cell lines in pre-clinical models，suppressing growth of xenografted tumor models（异种移植肿瘤模型）with FGFR alterations.

6. Initially，pemigatinib was evaluated in a phase Ⅰ/Ⅱ open-label study in a subset of patients with advanced solid tumors. In this study，pemigatinib was evaluated in three subsets of patients. Groups 1 and 3 had unselected advanced solid tumors and group 2 tumors harboring FGF/FGFR alteration. All patients with advanced solid tumors were refractory to prior therapy and had no further effective standard therapy.

7. Patients received pemigatinib orally once daily on a 21-day cycle（2-weeks on/1-week off）. In the dose escalation group 1，first 3 cohorts evaluated single patients and

subsequently a 3 + 3 design was used. In the dose expansion group 2, patients with FGFR rearrangements started on 9 mg once daily and increased to 13.5 mg once daily. In part 3 pemigatinib could be used in together with standard systemic therapies. Overall, about half of the patients presented hyperphosphatemia（高磷酸盐血）and fatigue, other adverse events observed included dry mouth, alopecia and stomatitis; most frequent grade ≥3 adverse events were pneumonia（10%）, fatigue（8%）, and hyponatremia（8%）. Hyperphosphatemia was easily managed with diet and phosphate binders; further dose modifications was also necessary. Based on preliminary safety and efficacy, the recommended phase Ⅱ dose selected was 13.5 mg once daily. In the dose expansion cohort, group 2, four patients with cholangiocarcinoma were treated with pemigatinib, with one achieving a partial response（PR）（部分响应）taking 9mg daily, with duration of response still ongoing at data cut-off.

8. The efficacy of pemigatinib in cholangiocarcinoma harboring FGFR alterations was further evaluated in the phase Ⅱ study FIGHT – 202. Patients with cholangiocarcinoma and disease progression after at least one previous treatment were assigned to one of three cohorts: patients with FGFR2-fusions or rearrangements, patients with other FGFR alterations, or patients with no FGFR alterations. The primary endpoint was objective response rate（ORR）（客观反应率）among those with fusions or rearrangements. From 1206 patients prescreened, a total of 146 patients were enrolled from multiple centers in USA, Europe, Middle East, and Asia; 107 patients had cholangiocarcinoma harboring fusions or rearrangements, 20 harbored other FGF/FGFR alterations, and 18 had no FGF/FGFR alterations. All patients received at least one dose of pemigatinib. After a median follow-up of 17.8 months, an ORR of 35.5% was observed in the 107 patients with fusions or rearrangements. Median PFS was 6.9 months and median OS was 21.1 months. No patients with other FGF/FGFR alterations achieved responses. The most common all-grade adverse event was hyperphosphatemia in 60% patients. Most frequent grade ≥3 adverse events were hypophosphatemia, arthralgia, stomatitis, hyponatremia, abdominal pain, and fatigue. Most frequent serious adverse events were abdominal pain, pyrexia, cholangitis, and pleural effusion. There were no treatment related deaths. Additionally, in another study, genomic analysis of patients who progressed on pemigatinib also revealed important information about this treatment. No statistical difference was observed in RR and PFS between cases classified as FGFR2-fusion versus rearranged. However, patients with co-occurring tumor suppression gene loss had shorter median PFS（p=0.000 3）.

9. Hyperphosphatemia is one of the most common adverse events related to FGFR inhibitors. It is an on-target effect related to FGFR inhibition. Multiple strategies are proposed to manage or prevent this adverse event, which includes dietary modifications, phosphate-lowering therapies（磷酸盐降低疗法）classified into

phosphate binders and phosphaturic agents and dose or schedule modifications. Available phosphate binders include magnesium hydroxide，calcium and iron-based regimens，lanthanum carbonate，and sevelamer.

10. Currently，an international phase Ⅲ randomized trial is recruiting patients to address pemigatinib against platinum-based chemotherapy as first-line therapy for unresectable or metastatic cholangiocarcinoma with FGFR2-fusions or rearrangements.

11. The FGFR inhibitor infigratinib（抑制剂英菲格拉替尼）was prospectively evaluated in patients with advanced cholangiocarcinoma with FGFR genomic alterations. In this phase Ⅱ study，a total of 61 patients were evaluated and treated with infigratinib 125 mg orally for 21 days of each 28-day cycle until unacceptable toxicity or disease progression. This result suggests that the efficacy of FGFR2 inhibitors may be higher in earlier lines of systemic treatment for advanced cholangiocarcinoma；ergo，studies evaluating these drugs on first-line setting might demonstrate higher benefit of these drugs.

From Frontiers in Oncology，2022，12（4）

After reading

Task 8　Build your vocabulary.

Directions：Match the following words with their corresponding definitions and Chinese equivalents.

English：heterogenous　malignance　cholangiocarcinoma　extrahepatic　inhibitor　escalation

Chinese：异基因的　恶性　胆管癌　肝外的　抑制剂　升级

Paras. 1—7

English	Chinese	Definition
1. _____	_____	a. consisting of elements that are not of the same kind or nature
2. _____	_____	b.（medicine）a malignant state
3. _____	_____	c. a kind of cancer
4. _____	_____	d. not closely related to liver
5. _____	_____	e. a substance which delays or prevents a chemical reaction
6. _____	_____	f. an increase to counteract a perceived discrepancy

Paras. 8—11

English: harbor alteration abdominal adverse dietary stomatitis

Chinese: 怀有 改变 腹部的 不利的 饮食中的 口炎

English	Chinese	Definition
7. _____	_____	g. maintain（a theory，thoughts，or feelings）
8. _____	_____	h. a change to sth that makes it different
9. _____	_____	i. relating to or connected with the abdomen
10. _____	_____	j. negative and unpleasant；not likely to produce a good result
11. _____	_____	k. substances such as fibre and fat that are found in food
12. _____	_____	l. inflammation of the mucous membrane of the mouth

Guiding to learn

Task 9   Learn the following general academic vocabulary from the word bank.

assessment variant complex consequently evaluation impact regulation
contribute demonstrate ensure framework outcome proportion sequence access
confer emerging implementation integrate mechanism statistically capacity
compounded exposure facilitate modification modifying precision stabilize
welfare diverse initiate transform dynamic complement highlight intensify
predominantly prospective mediate depression likewise ongoing

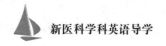

Beginning to read

Task 10   Now read the text.

Text C

Delivering Paediatric Precision Medicine: Genomic and Environmental Considerations along the Causal Pathway of Childhood Neurodevelopmental Disorders

Sue Woolfenden et al

1. Precision medicine refers to treatments that are tailored or targeted to the needs of the individual based on their genetic, biomarker, phenotypic, and/or psychosocial characteristics. While having an established history in fields such as paediatric oncology(儿科肿瘤学), with a focus on identifying specific biological mechanisms and molecular pathways to provide specific treatment recommendations and improve outcomes in childhood cancer, precision medicine is increasingly being applied across other paediatric fields, including for children with neurodevelopmental disorders. Globally it has been estimated that there are 53 million children and young people who have a neurodevelopmental disorder. They have a range of diverse symptoms and syndromes related to problems of neurodevelopment including epilepsy, common monogenic neurological disorders(常见的单基因神经系统疾病), rare genetic disorders, intellectual disability, cerebral palsy, autism spectrum disorder, Tourette syndrome, obsessive-compulsive disorder, and attention-deficit/ hyperactivity disorder. Although children and young people with neurodevelopmental disorders show great resilience across the life course, they are more likely to have higher levels of physical and mental health morbidity and mortality, are less likely to complete education, and are more likely to be unemployed and be socially isolated. This not only results in a poorer quality of life for the individual but also a loss of productivity and increased health and welfare expenditure costs at a societal level. In this narrative review we aim to highlight the current challenges and the therapeutic potential of precision medicine in neurodevelopmental disorders(神经发育障碍). We present a biopsychosocial integrated framework to examine the "gene-environment neuroscience interaction"(神经科学的基因和环境互动). We highlight the need for the power of big data, transdiagnostic assessment, impact and implementation evaluation, and a bench-to-bedside scientific discovery agenda with ongoing clinician and patient engagement.

2. Recently，precision medicine for neurodevelopmental disorders has predominantly harnessed advances in genomic sequencing technologies to increase our ability to identify single gene mutations（单基因突变），diagnose a multitude of rare neurodevelopmental disorders，and gain insights into pathogenesis. There have been clear successes in the application of such a precision medicine approach to monogenic neurodevelopmental disorders. Paediatric monogenic neurological disorders affect around 1% of children at birth，and neurological disorders in general are the primary cause of disability in global burden of disease analysis. For those with monogenic disorders，early molecular diagnosis is important for genetic counselling and patient management.

3. Spinal muscular atrophy（脊髓性肌肉萎缩）is an exemplar of a monogenic neurodevelopmental disorder，in which identifying and understanding the genetic underpinnings has driven development and clinical translation of genetic therapies across the spectrum of phenotypes，together with population screening imperatives to prevent and mitigate disease burden. This has especially transformed the lives of young children with spinal muscular atrophy，who no longer have a condition with progressive decline in motor function，with presymptomatic infants treated with disease modifying therapies attaining independent walking. Consequently，newborn screening programmes for spinal muscular atrophy have been implemented and welcomed by families and health professionals alike，to improve equitable care，and optimize outcomes and cost-effectiveness. Likewise，robust clinical trial pipelines targeting multiple physiological pathways to safely reduce progression，stabilize，or improve function across diverse neuromuscular disorders are emerging，including Charcot—Marie—Tooth disease，congenital myasthenic syndromes（先天性肌无力综合征），muscular dystrophies（肌肉营养不良），and congenital myopathies.

3. Although advances continue to be made for monogenic neurodevelopmental disorders，the diagnostic yield of whole exome or genome sequencing（全外显子组或基因组测序）depends upon the disorder. Disruptions in more than 900 different genes that contribute to brain development and function are reported among neurodevelopmental disorders. 11 Examples of the diagnostic yield of genomic testing found the proportion of patients with a "monogenic" cause of their neurodevelopmental disorder varies by the diagnostic category. Notably，some studies target recruitment of high-risk subpopulations and thus the diagnostic yield for the total population may be lower than reported in these tables. So，while for some neurodevelopmental disorders，such as intellectual disability，advances in next generation sequencing technologies have increased diagnostic yield to more than 40%，this is not the case for many neurodevelopmental disorders that are common including attention-deficit/hyperactivity disorder，obsessive-compulsive disorder（强迫症），Tourette's syndrome（图雷特氏综合征），and autism spectrum disorder（自闭症谱系障

碍). Furthermore, a confirmed genetic diagnosis in a neurodevelopmental disorder will only provide an effective targeted "precision" treatment, such as vitamin supplementation, cofactor, enzyme replacement, pharmacological or genetic therapies for less than 10% of individuals at present. A monogenic diagnosis does however enable prospective reproductive decision-making for parents, facilitated through genetic counselling. While common genetic variants have been identified as important and cumulative contributors to their pathogenesis as outlined in Table S2, most children with neurodevelopmental disorders are likely to have multiple genes with small contributions, so gene therapy may not address their therapeutic needs, even in the future. This highlights the need for a broader conceptualization of precision medicine in neurodevelopmental disorders.

From Developmental Medicine & Child Neurology, *2022*, *64*(*9*)

New words and expressions

phenotypic /ˌfiːnəˈtɪpɪk/ *adj*. of or relating to or constituting a phenotype 表(现)型的

paediatric /ˌpiːdɪˈætrɪk/ *adj*. of or relating to the medical care of children 儿科的

oncology /ɒŋˈkɒlədʒi/ *n*. the scientific study of and treatment of tumors in the body 肿瘤学

monogenic /ˌmɒnəʊˈdʒenɪk/ *adj*. of or relating to an inheritable character that is controlled by a single pair of genes 单基因的,单性生殖的

hyperactivity /ˌhaɪpərækˈtɪvəti/ *n*. a condition characterized by excessive restlessness and movement 机能亢进

morbidity /mɔːˈbɪdɪti/ *n*. the quality of being unhealthful and generally bad for you 发病率;病态

expenditure /ɪkˈspendɪtʃə(r)/ *n*. the use of energy, time, materials, etc. (精力、时间、材料等的)耗费,消耗

syndromes /ˈsɪndrəʊmz/ *n*. a medical condition that is characterized by a particular group of signs and symptoms 综合征;综合症状

sub-population /ˈsʌbpɒpjʊˈleɪʃən/ *n*. a population that is part of a larger population 子总体;亚种群

compulsive /kəmˈpʌlsɪv/ *adj*. that is difficult to stop or control 难以制止的;难控制的

pharmacological /ˌfɑːməkəˈlɒdʒɪkl/ *adj*. of or relating to pharmacology 药理学的

conceptualization /kənˌseptjʊəlaɪˈzeɪʃən/ *n*. inventing or contriving an idea or explanation and formulating it mentally 化为概念,概念化

crosstalk /ˈkrɒstɔːk/ *n*. a situation in which a communications system is picking up the wrong signals 串话,串扰

perinatal /ˌperɪˈneɪtl/ *adj*. at or around the time of birth 临产的;围产期的

After reading

Task 11   **Build your vocabulary. Choose one word which can be used to replace the language shown in bold without changing the meaning of the sentence from the list below. Change forms and cases when necessary.**

accomplish (*v.*)   adequate (*adj.*)   area (*n.*)   chemical (*adj.*)   conduct (*v.*) consume (*v.*)   credible (*adj.*)   dispose of (*v.*)   exert (*v.*)   manifest (*v.*) occupy (*v.*)   rely on (*v.*)

1. It is still the direction that government and citizens should work together to reduce plastic littering, and to guide people not to **throw away** plastic rubbish in the soil environment.   _____

2. SHS contains a complex mixture of 4000 **substances** including known fetal developmental toxicants.   _____

3. In addition to these dispositions, we suggest that perceptions of the facilitator as **plausible**, relatable, and likable are implicit drivers of participant engagement and receptiveness to intervention messages.   _____

4. To truly curb HIV incidence among YMSM, we can not solely **depend on** one strategy to prevent and treat HIV.   _____

5. Previous studies have shown a significant increase in local recurrence rates after 1 cm excisions, suggesting that 1 cm margins might not be **sufficient** to deal with local microsatellitosis.   _____

6. Although such patients are uncommon, they cause a significant disruption and danger to the ED and **use** time and resources required for other patients.

    _____

7. Fragmentation, adaptor ligation, and index ligation were **achieved** using the Nextera XT DNA Sample Preparation Kit (Illumina) following the recommended protocol.   _____

8. Most importantly, genomic sequences **filled** by IkBalpha essentially overlapped with those regions containing high H3K27me3 levels (Figure 3G).

    _____

9. There is now firm evidence that bilirubin **exercises** strong antioxidant activities in mammals, which have been mainly attributed to its active role of efficient scavenger of reactive oxygen species (ROS).   _____

10. Thus, the primary aim of this study was to investigate resumption of puberty as **shown** by menarche in girls and testicular volume increase in boys after histrelin explantation in a diverse group of patients with and without CPP.

    _____

Further reading

Abdelhalim，H.，Berber，A.，Lodi，M.，et al.（2022）. Artificial Intelligence，Healthcare，Clinical Genomics，and Pharmacogenomics Approaches in Precision Medicine. *Front Genet*. 13(6).

Carrasco-Ramiro，F.，Peiró-Pastor，R.，Aguado，B.（2017）. Human Genomics Projects and Precision Medicine. *Gene Therapy*. 24(9).

Woolfenden，S.，Farrar，M. A.，Eapen，V.，et al.（2022）. Delivering Paediatric Precision Medicine：Genomic and Environmental Considerations along the Causal Pathway of Childhood Neurodevelopmental Disorders. *Developmental Medicine & Child Neurology*. 64(9).

Zugman，M.，Botrus，G.，Pestana，R. C.，et al.（2022）. Precision Medicine Targeting FGFR2 Genomic Alterations in Advanced Cholangiocarcinoma：Current State and Future Perspectives. *Frontiers in Oncology*. 12(4).

Unit 4
Accurate Immunology

Guiding to learn

Several conceptual pillars form the foundation of modern immunology. The intersection of immunology and nanotechnology has provided significant advancements in biomedical research and clinical applications over the years. Neurosurgery as one of the most technologically demanding medical fields rapidly adapts the newest developments from multiple scientific disciplines for treating brain tumors. Zinc homeostasis is vital for functioning of the immune and other organs and systems.

Discuss the following questions with your partners.

1. What are achievements of nanomedicine and immunology?
2. What is Zinc homeostasis?
3. What is your understanding of immunology?

Task 1   Learn the following general academic vocabulary.

acquire administration impact normal potentially previously component contribute conventional correspond criteria emphasize initial maximize outcome volume promoter retention challenge entity exposure facilitate modify enhance gender incorporate   minimum comprise accumulation complement eventually induce minimize thereby encounter

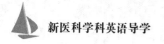

Beginning to read

Task 2　Now read the text.

Text A

Neurosurgery at the Crossroads of Immunology and Nanotechnology
Vladimir A. Ljubimov et al

1. The term "nano neurosurgery"（纳米神经外科）is less than two decades old. In 2003，Dunn and Black for the first time proposed it to use for glioma therapies（神经胶质瘤治疗）on a molecular scale. Nanomaterials for nano neurosurgery as imaging and treatment agents are selected for a number of criteria corresponding to the "brain rules"：1）Neuroprotection and lack of neurotoxicity，2）Ability to be delivered through BBB，3）Pharmacological criteria，which are prolongation of plasma circulation，tumor accumulation and cancer cell retention，4）specific targeting of a brain cell type，5）Immunomodulation of the brain privileged immune system，and 6）Resensitization to the other treatment's effects.

2. The tendency in modern neurosurgery is to minimize surgical invasiveness by incorporating novel imaging techniques and personalized surgical and treatment approaches. The theranostic approach，that is，the ability to deliver imaging and therapeutic agents to the tumor site and tumor cells using one nano agent hold great promise. Molecular imaging with the development of long term circulating and targeting agents expands the options for both diagnostic and therapeutical strategies. Nano-pharmacology in this setting allows for systemic drug administration to enhance drug concentrations in the tumors to maximize efficacy and minimize systemic and neuro toxicity（神经毒性）. Nanotechnology may address a number of needs at the same time through the design of multifunctional agents able to act in the myriad of combinations of targeted and immune-therapeutical agents often needed to eradicate the existing tumors and prevent tumor growth and recurrence.

3. Development and optimization of effective delivery methods of nanoplatforms may significantly improve the treatment of malignant gliomas（恶性胶质瘤）and other brain tumors in the near future. This is achieved through facilitating in vivo therapeutic targeting of tumor endothelial system and parenchymal cells（实质细胞），thereby permitting access to the tumor microenvironment and its component immune system. With the advent of "nano neurosurgery"，targeted and efficient molecular therapeutics and immunotherapy would soon complement the current surgical，

radiological，and chemotherapeutic approaches to the management of diseases in neurooncology.

4. This review discusses achievements of nanomedicine and immunology that could improve brain tumor treatment. Specifically，we focus on the clinical translation toward precision medicine to improve patient-specific therapeutic responses (患者特异性的治疗反应). We emphasize new biomaterials，drugs and bioengineering approaches aimed to overcome biological barriers and individual tumor heterogeneity. The classes and subclasses of nanomaterials that are currently under development or used in clinic for brain imaging and therapy are presented with evaluation of their physico-chemical properties that correspond to the clinical needs.

5. Precision medicine，or personalized medicine，calls for the development of patient-tailored treatments (病人量身定制的治疗) based on biomarkers or stratification by mutations or biomarkers. While not yet a clinical reality，the premise of precision medicine is that it will offer superior outcomes to the traditional treatment of disease rather than a one-treatment-per-disease approach to cancer management. Patient stratification has already become a standard for new drug development，because anti-cancer therapeutics often show little efficacy in unstratified studies.

6. Although patient stratification is essential in the development of precision medicines，clinical trials for nanodrugs are currently conducted in unstratified populations. This situation may soon change，as the importance of stratification becomes more obvious，and nanodrugs begin to gear toward specific patient populations. Nanodrugs can circumvent many current problems of delivery，which may potentially improve therapeutic efficacy of precision medicines. This may also allow more patients to receive individualized therapies.

7. Gliomas are the most common primary malignant brain tumors(恶性脑肿瘤)，comprising around 75% of all primary malignant brain tumors in adults. Of various gliomas，glioblastoma is the most prevalent and the most lethal. The precise etiology of GBM is unknown，and the prevalence of GBMs is projected to increase as the population ages. This may be due to increases in exposure to ionizing radiation and environmental factors that induce inflammation，as well as other sources of genomic insults. Gliomas appear to be sex-dependent，with males having around 1.6fold higher probability of acquiring this pathology than do females. In addition，females have a better response to therapy. The exact cause of sex dependence is not clear. A recent study has found molecular differences in gliomas depending on gender and suggests the need of further research to unravel their significance and potentially modify the treatment. Gliomas of low grades（Ⅰ-Ⅱ）have a higher survival rate，although all gliomas including high grades（Ⅲ-Ⅳ）eventually result in death. The conventional standard of treatment including surgery followed by radiation and chemotherapy is decades old and only results in a modest survival benefit. The combination treatment

using temozolomide（TMZ）（替莫唑胺）with radiation therapy has led to a significant increase in patient survival rates. Tumor resection is one of the primary treatment methods，though many risk factors may impact the patient's outcome，and prevention of novel neurological deficits as a result of tumor resection is placed at a higher value than the resection itself. While majority of cases of initial recurrence are in or in the vicinity of resection in patients with GBM，late recurrences typically involve diffuse infiltrating disease distant from site of origin and not easily amenable to surgical therapy.

8. Several known biomarkers，such as O6-methylguanine-DNA methyltransferase （MGMT）methylation and isocitrate dehydrogenase（IDH）（异柠檬酸脱氢酶）have been identified in terms of stratifying glioma response. Reduced MGMT protein expression regulated by its promoter methylation helps prevent cellular apoptosis（细胞凋亡）caused by TMZ treatment. Therefore，tumor susceptibility to TMZ treatment is increased. Additionally，IDH mutations are present in many secondary GBM tumors，and in around 10% of all gliomas. As of 2021，the updated WHO CNS tumor classification separates IDH mutated GBM as different astrocytoma grade II-IV. IDH mutated GBMs are their own separate entity and are grade IV. Despite advances in cancer therapy，treatment of GBM remains a significant challenge due to the paucity of curative options. One major hurdle is the inability of anticancer drugs to efficiently traverse the blood-brain barrier（BBB）（血脑屏障）to reach the tumor cells. Therefore，novel drug delivery methods that can easily cross the BBB and deliver anticancer drugs to tumor cells without affecting normal cells are desired. It is hoped that Nanotechnology and nanoimmunology may significantly contribute to the future treatment of gliomas by facilitating BBB traversal to allow for novel brain cancer treatments，including both direct targeting of the tumor and perhaps in combination with immunotherapy.

9. In addition to common primary brain tumors like GBM，a more rare and similarly deadly primary brain tumor is primary central nervous system lymphoma （PCNSL）（原发性中枢神经系统淋巴瘤）. Lymphomas are hematologic malignancies（恶性血液病）developing from lymphocytes. Within the four groups of non-Hodgkin lymphomas（NHL）（非霍奇金氏淋巴瘤）there are over 60 specific types of tumors. Lymphomas are considered as immunologically "hot" tumors，which will respond to immunotherapy. It was interesting to compare the PCNSL treatment response with other tumors，e.g.，GBM，that are "cold" and do not respond easily to all kinds of immune stimulations. PCNSL represents only 4% to 6% of all extranodal lymphomas，but its incidence among immunocompetent patients is increasing，particularly among persons 65 years of age and older. This problem is getting more important nowadays with tendency to increasing longevity and geriatric population. Men are twice as likely to acquire this pathology than women. PCNSL is encountered in the brain，eyes，and

cerebrospinal fluid（CSF）（脑脊髓液）but has no systemic manifestations，similar to the other brain primary glial tumor，GBM. About 95% of PCNSLs are diffuse large B-cell lymphomas that are typically highly infiltrative neoplasms，characterized as a "whole brain disease"，particularly at relapse. Like malignant gliomas，PCNSL is not amenable to curative resection. For treated lymphomas located outside the CNS，the 5-year survival is 67%—79%. However，treated PCNSL patients have 5-year survival rate of only 20%—25%. At present，there is no standard treatment for recurrent PCNSL.

From Advanced Drug Delivery Reviews，2022，181（2）

New words and expressions

neurosurgery /ˌnjʊərəʊˈsɜːdʒəri/ *n*. operations on any part of the nervous system including the brain，spinal cord，and individual nerves 神经外科手术

eradicate /ɪˈrædɪkeɪt/ *vt*. to destroy or get rid of sth completely，as if down to the roots 根除；根绝；消灭

heterogeneity /ˌhetərəˈdʒəˈniːəti/ *n*. the quality of being diverse and not comparable in kind 多相性；异质性

stratification /ˌstrætɪfɪˈkeɪʃən/ *n*. forming or depositing in layers 分层；成层法

circumvent /ˌsɜːkəmˈvent/ *vt*. avoid or try to avoid fulfilling，answering，or performing (duties，questions，or issues) 规避；设法避开

diffuse /dɪˈfjuːs/ *vt*. (cause to) spread out freely in all directions 扩散；散开

amenable /əˈmiːnəbl/ *adj*. disposed or willing to comply 顺从的；易控制的

geriatric /ˌdʒeriˈætrɪk/ *adj*. of or relating to the aged 老年医学的；老人的

infiltrative /ˈɪnfɪltrətɪv/ *adj*. spreading gradually to affect all parts of a place or thing 渗透性的；造成渗透的

nanotechnology /ˌnænəʊtekˈnɒlədʒi/ *n*. the branch of engineering that deals with things smaller than 100 nanometers (especially with the manipulation of individual molecules) 纳米技术

polymeric /ˌpɒliˈmerɪk/ *adj*. of or relating to or consisting of a polymer 聚合的；聚合物的

inorganic /ˌɪnɔːˈgænɪk/ *adj*. relating or belonging to the class of compounds not having a carbon basis 无机的；非自然生长的

nucleic acid /njuːˌkliːɪkˈæsɪd/ any of various macromolecules composed of nucleotide chains that are vital constituents of all living cells 核酸

cerebrospinal fluid clear liquid produced in the ventricles of the brain 脑脊髓液

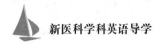

After reading

Task 3　Read Text A again and answer the following questions.

1. How much do you know about nanotechnology?

2. What's the function of nanotechnology?

Task 4　Check your vocabulary. Fill in the blanks with the correct form of the words from the following box, each word can be used only once.

impress(*v.*)	energy(*n.*)	distribute(*v.*)	speculate(*v.*)	assemble(*v.*)	reject(*v.*)
analogy(*n.*)	spontaneous(*adj.*)	perpendicular(*adj.*)	text(*n.*)	administer(*v.*)	
intervene(*v.*)					

1. I find a flaw in the _____ in that the two metaphysics describe the same events, but the two theories do not.

2. The lush green meadows of the valley, enhanced by the Paiute, _____ white explorers and accounts of the valley remarked on its potential for settlement and agriculture.

3. At the same time, they may be aware that they are _____ by American society (e.g. discrimination), and they may be afraid of displeasing their parents who may want their children to maintain their cultural roots and values.

4. This type of model would result in creative inventions that were both _____ and practical.

5. Peters discusses throughout the _____ about how the world is changing and everything will be completely re-invented within the next 25 years.

6. In essence, T2 measures decay of magnetization _____ to the main magnetic field.

7. Since corporations are only concerned with profit, the government must _____ to provide a standard of health and nutrition for consumers.

8. He is channeling _____ into doing something constructive and helpful for his family instead of engaging in other more unacceptable behaviors.

9. The criteria for sex discrimination under Title VII that sexual harassment researchers are most familiar with have been _____ across multiple court cases.

10. If this intervention were to be redone, there would be significant benefits to having a handout that could be _____ to each individual student.

Task 5　Build your vocabulary. Read the sentences below, decide which word in each bracket is more suitable.

1. Greater contribution to the finances of the family, spatial mobility and access to social and economic resources beyond the domestic (sphere/globe), provide females with greater leverage in their appeals for even greater autonomy and independence.

2. Moreover, as a student in clinical (psychology/biology), I could not avoid thinking about what clinical psychologists can and should do in the process of prevention and intervention.

3. An independent samples t-test was conducted to (assess/investigate) whether the categorical variable gender and the continuous variable measured by the constructs of the students' participation in class are associated.

4. They are conceived of as far down the vertical inner (axis/axle) that extends from every objective event, to the point where they are consigned to a different Earth.

5. Central to his argument is how race serves as a "master status-determining characteristic" that overrides the individual identity of any given black man in the mind of the stranger who (praises/appraises) them.

6. One process that differentiates speech processing from reading is the process of phonological recoding, or of mapping specific phonemes onto visual (shapes/symbols).

7. The collective unconscious is not dependent on cerebral (heredity/inheritance); it is the result of what I shall call the unreflected imposition of a culture...It is normal for the Antillean to be anti-Negro.

8. Naturally, then, forest dwellers are prominent subjects of (discourse/chat) on conservation in India, and their interests are most strongly affected by conservation policies and measures.

9. However, children can also (acquire/obtain) positive skills from television viewing.

10. Some (approximate/tentative) database I will turn to are ICPSR, UM China Data Center and National Statistical Bureau of China.

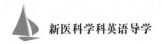
新医科学科英语导学

Guiding to learn

Task 6　Learn the following general academic vocabulary.

distribution percentage process variant complex alternative consent layer maximum shift implicate mechanism resolution statistical status summarize undertake capacity index transport utilise channel convert automatically induce intensity uniform analogous ethics mediate medium protocol supplement panel undergoing

Beginning to read

Task 7　Now read the text.

Text B

Immunolocalization of Zinc Transporters and Metallothioneins Reveals Links to Microvascular Morphology and Functions
Hai B. Tran et al

1. The complex system of small blood vessels, namely arterioles, capillaries and venules, collectively called microvessels, is central in life-threatening conditions such as pulmonary arterial hypertension（PAH）（肺动脉高压）, coronary microvascular disease（冠状动脉微血管疾病） and microvascular brain disease（微血管性脑病）. The microvascular wall consists of a few cell types, of which endothelial and smooth muscle cells are the two major populations in arterioles and venules. In healthy adult microvessels, both these cell types are relatively quiescent, not proliferating, but sensitive to chemical or mechanical stimuli for activation. This activation may lead to increased cell proliferation and even switching of the smooth muscle cell phenotype, resulting in a broad range of morphological and physiological changes known as "vascular remodelling"（血管重构）. In animal models of diabetes and metabolic syndrome, hypertrophic remodelling of microvessels was identified in early stages when coronary arteries remained normal by angiography, indicating a key role for

58

remodelling of micro-rather than macrovessels in initiation of haemodynamic disorders in these disease.

2. Zinc homeostasis is vital for functioning of the immune and other organs and systems. Cellular zinc homeostasis is regulated by three major families of proteins: (1) Solute Carrier 39 family/Zrt-and Irt-like proteins, which import zinc ions into the cytosolic compartment from the extracellular space or intracellular vesicles; (2) Solute Carrier 30 family/Zinc transporters, which export zinc ions from the cytosolic compartment to the extracellular space, or intracellular vesicles; (3) Metallothioneins (MTs)(金属硫蛋白), which have a high zinc binding capacity, thus playing key roles in intracellular zinc storage and buffering. To date, 14 ZIPs, 10 ZnTs and 4 isoforms of MTs with multiple subtypes/variants have been described in mammals.

3. ZIPs have been identified as playing major roles in a broad array of vital functions and diseases. Their expression and functional roles in vascular physiology and diseases had been paid little attention until the recent ground-breaking finding that ZIP12 is at least partly responsible for hypoxia-induced PAH in both human and rats, inspiring other studies into this field. Data on vascular expression and functions of other members of the zinc regulation system remain scant. ZIP14 was shown to mediate infux of $Zn2+$ in sheep pulmonary artery endothelial cells, which may act together with MT to protect against LPS-induced apoptosis. MT expression and anti-oxidative stress functions in vasculature have been implicated in a number of studies using models of cultured endothelial cells. Thus, despite a growing interest into the zinc regulation system in vascular health and diseases, the understanding of vascular expression and functions of ZIPs, ZnTs and MTs in vivo remains a large gap in our knowledge. A systematic background analysis of the zinc regulation system in human vasculature would benefit further investigations in this field.

4. Following on from our previous study aiming to characterize the zinc regulation system in human vasculature, in this study we employed multifuorescence quantitative confocal microscopy (MQCM)(多荧光定量共聚焦显微镜) to investigate immunoreactivities of human microvessels in paraffin tissue sections for multiple ZIPs and MTs. Their detailed distribution among the major cell types of microvessels and association with microvascular morphology and expression of vascular function-related molecules was investigated.

Materials and methods
Antibodies

5. A panel of 13 primary antibodies to zinc transporters and metallothioneins and 6 to other molecules was used in this study. Their source, animal species, class/type, dilutions, immunogens and published details relating to specificity are summarized in Supporting Information.

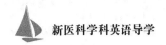

6. To minimize cross reactivity in multifuorescence labeling（多重前缀标签），all secondary antibodies were donkey IgG F（ab）2 fragments，absorbed against cross-species reactivities. They were obtained from Jackson ImmunoResearch，including anti-rabbit IgG-AF594，anti-goat IgG-AF488 and anti-mouse IgG-AF647，used at 1∶200. For alternative combinations of primary antibodies in some experiments conjugates switched colours.

Human tissue samples

8. Subcutaneous tissue biopsies（皮下组织活检）were collected from 14 patients undergoing hernia reconstructive surgeries at The Queen Elizabeth Hospital in Adelaide，Australia. Informed consent was obtained from each donor，utilising protocols approved by the Central Adelaide Local Health Network Human Research Ethics Committee at The Queen Elizabeth Hospital. According to the ethics approval，individual patient demographic data and their disease status were known only to three authors，RJ，JB and PZ.

Tissue processing and histology

9. To minimize variations that could have resulted from tissue processing，the pre-fixation time when tissue samples were preserved in RPMI medium on ice for transport was kept ＜ 2 h；the fixation protocol was kept uniformly for 24 h at room temperature in phosphate saline-buffered 10% formalin，a protocol accepted by most authors. For quantitative analysis，sections from multiple paraffin blocks were cut to 5 μm thickness and mounted onto tissue arrays for batch analysis of all samples.

10. Tissue sections were stained with H&E in a standard protocol at the Histopathology service at Adelaide Health and Medical Sciences and then scanned at a 40×objective with a Nanozoomer digital slide scanner.

Multifuorescence quantitative confocal microscopy (MQCM)

11. Immunofluorescence of human paraffin tissue sections was performed following a protocol described in our previous study. MQCM was carried out using an Olympus confocal microscopy system and ImageJ morphometric software as previously described. Briefly，ten optical fields containing microvessels were serially captured from each biopsy under a 60 × silicone immersed objective simultaneously in four fluorescence channels set for AF488，AF594，AF647 and DAPI. All microvessels of 20—100 μm diameter in each frame were then selected and their areas in monochromatic images measured for mean fluorescence intensities（MFI）（平均荧光强度）by Image J. Analogous to the flow cytometry mean fluorescence intensity（MFI），which is a quantitative measurement of fluorescence brightness averaged from all events counted in a gate，in immunofluorescence MFI is averaged from all pixels of the

region of interest（ROI）of an image. MFI values were measured using MQCM as follows. From a merged multi-colour confocal image, the area of a microvessel section as the ROI was delineated first using the Image J software drawing tools. Using the CTR-SHIFT-E keys, the ROI was then applied to monochromatic channel images which had previously been converted to greyscale by menu Image/Type/16-bit. Then, the menu Image/Adjust/Threshold was applied, allowing the software to automatically predict a threshold. Next, in the menu Analyze/Analyze Particles, the mean greyvalue was selected from Set Measurement to measure the ROI MFI. The MFIs of ten ROIs captured from each sample were averaged and corrected for autofluorescent background. The latter were measured for each channel in a similar way as for the samples stained with conjugate alone（negative controls, which were included in every batch analysis）. For punctate immunofuorescence of ET－1, particle counting function was carried out in a predetermined threshold band for uniform gating in only bright particle sizing of$>$10 square pixels（>3.13 μm^2）. Numbers of particles counted in a vascular area were then normalized by numbers of nuclei counted in the DAPI channel in the same area.

12. Microvessels were subdivided into two subpopulations, "muscularized" when having walls consisting of at least two cell layers in the whole perimeter and "non-muscularized" for walls consisting of fewer than two layers. The percentage of "muscularized" microvessels varied between 0 and $\sim$60%.

13. After obtaining quantitative results of all included samples, representative confocal images were selected for those most closely reflecting the final quantitative results, without referring to the donor age and disease status.

14. Statistical analysis was undertaken using Prism 9 software（GraphPad Software, CA, USA）. For difference between subgroups of microvessels, a paired two-tailed Wilcoxon test was used. Changes were considered statistically significant at $p<0.05$.

From Histochemistry and Cell Biology, 2022, 158(5)

After reading

Task 8   Build your vocabulary.

Directions: Match the following words with their corresponding definitions and Chinese equivalents.

Paras. 1—8

English：quiescent proliferating vascular conjugate protocol variation simultaneously monochromatic

Chinese：结合 增殖的 变异 单色的 血管的 协议 静止状态的 同时发生

English	Chinese	Definition
1._____	_____	a. rules determining the format and transmission of data
2._____	_____	b. unite chemically so that the product is easily broken down into the original compounds
3._____	_____	c. not developing，especially when this is probably only a temporary state
4._____	_____	d. of or relating to or having vessels that conduct and circulate fluids
5._____	_____	e. cause to grow or increase rapidly
6._____	_____	f. having or appearing to have only one color
7._____	_____	g. at the same instant
8._____	_____	h. an instance of change

Paras. 9—14

English：subdivide perimeter demographic pathological cardiovascular scatter demarcate

Chinese：病理学的 周长 心血管的 人口统计的 再分 区别 散布

English	Chinese	Definition
9._____	_____	i. caused by or evidencing a mentally disturbed condition
10._____	_____	j. the size of something as given by the distance around it
11._____	_____	k. a statistic characterizing human populations
12._____	_____	l. a haphazard distribution in all directions
13._____	_____	m. divide into smaller and smaller pieces
14._____	_____	n. of or pertaining to or involving the heart and blood vessels
15._____	_____	o. separate clearly and as if by boundaries

Guiding to learn

Task 9   Learn the following general academic vocabulary from the word bank.

beneficial   function issue   distinct   illustration mechanism   sustaining neutralize

adaptive   trigger   encounter

Beginning to read

Task 10   Now read the text.

Text C

Nanomaterials in Immunology: Bridging Innovative Approaches in Immune Modulation, Diagnostics, and Therapy

George-Alexandru Croitoru et al

1. Immunology is the science that studies all the functions of the immune system (免疫系统), or immunity. The immune system is the body's defense mechanism against harmful microorganisms (like bacteria, fungi, and viruses) and protects it against infections and diseases. The immune system consists of a complex network of cells, tissues, and organs, such as bone marrow (骨髓), skin, spleen, and mucous membranes (黏膜), and it recognizes and neutralizes the intruders while protecting the healthy cells and organs. It is divided into innate immunity and adaptive immunity (先天免疫和适应性免疫), both of which have roles in sustaining the body's health and protecting it against disease. Innate immunity provides the first defense mechanism, and it consists of four protective barriers: (a) physical barriers, such as skin and mucous membranes; (b) physiologic barriers (生理屏障), which involve temperature and chemical mediators; (c) endocytic/phagocytic, where specific cells uptake the foreign microorganism; (d) inflammatory, involving the recruitment of different cells (such as macrophages). A schematic illustration (示意图) of innate immunity's barriers is presented in Figure 1. Adaptive immunity is the second defense mechanism, and it involves specialized cells, more precisely lymphocytes, that remember and respond

more effectively to previously encountered pathogens. Adaptive immunity can be slower than the innate one, but after it fights off one type of pathogen, it will be eradicated much faster the next time it is encountered. The adaptive immunity system is made of B cells and T cells, two distinct groups of lymphocytes and antibodies, and all are responsible for the immune responses.

2. There has been a growing interest in combining immunology with nanotechnology in the past few years. This multidisciplinary area of study focuses on creating materials at the nanoscale (纳米级) to control and understand immunological reactions (免疫反应). A few challenges and aims currently exist in immunology, including developing new diagnostic methods and treatments for immune diseases and improving immune responses to vaccines and infections. These shortcomings can be addressed by using nanotechnology. Specifically, overcoming these issues involves using nanomaterials, materials between 1 and 100 nm with unique properties such as small size, shape, and structure, which can be modified to fit the desired use. These materials can be designed to modulate immune functions by interacting with immune cells. Nanomaterials could be applied in the field of immunology by being used as carriers for drugs, antigens (抗原), or nucleic acids (核酸).

3. Researchers aim to improve medical procedures, like diagnostics and treatments in immunology, with the help of nanomaterials. Because of their small size and high area-to-volume ratio, therapeutic drugs can be loaded more efficiently and in higher quantities, resulting in effective delivery to specific cells or tissues. This leads to an increased therapeutic effect and reduced side effects because only diseased cells are targeted without affecting healthy ones. Nanomaterials have promising effects that can make them suitable for diagnostics. Researchers aim to create extremely specific and sensitive biosensors (生物传感器) that can identify biomarkers at low concentrations, making early diagnosis possible, which could improve patient outcomes in future applications. For instance, pathogens or proteins linked to disease can be precisely captured and detected using nanoparticles (NPs) (纳米颗粒) linked with antibodies or other ligands.

4. Nanomaterials have mainly demonstrated their beneficial effects in treating autoimmune diseases and cancer, among other immune-related conditions. Immunomodulatory drugs (免疫调节药物) can be directly delivered to immune cells via NPs, changing their activity and improving the body's natural immunological response. In cancer therapy, nanomaterials can be used to deliver chemotherapeutic (化学疗法的) drugs directly to tumors, so the damage to healthy cells is reduced and the therapeutic effect is improved.

5. Nanomaterials can cross biological barriers like the blood - brain barrier (血脑屏障), thereby creating alternative treatments for neurological diseases. Furthermore, nanomaterials show promise in more durable vaccine development because they may

trigger prolonged immune responses.

From Journal of Functional Biomaterials，*2024*，*15（8）*

New words and expressions

immunology /ˌɪmjuˈnɒlədʒi/ *n*. the branch of medical science that studies the body's immune system 免疫学

immunity /ɪˈmjuːnəti/ *n*. the body's ability to avoid or not be affected by infection and disease 免疫力

microorganism /ˌmaɪkrəʊˈɔːgənɪzəm/ *n*. any organism of microscopic size 微生物；微小动植物

fungi /ˈfʌŋiː/ *n*. the taxonomic kingdom of lower plants 真菌；菌类；蘑菇（fungus 的复数）

spleen /spliːn/ *n*. a small organ near the stomach that controls the quality of the blood cells 脾脏；坏脾气；怒气

phagocytic /ˌfægəˈsɪtɪk/ *adj*. capable of functioning as a phagocyte 噬菌作用的；噬菌细胞的

inflammatory /ɪnˈflæmət(ə)ri/ *adj*. causing or involving inflammation 发炎的；炎性的

lymphocyte /ˈlɪmfəʊˌsaɪt/ *n*. an agranulocytic leukocyte that normally makes up a quarter of the white blood cell count but increases in the presence of infection 淋巴球

pathogen /ˈpæθədʒən/ *n*. a thing that causes disease 病原体

vaccine /ˈvæksiːn/ *n*. immunogen consisting of a suspension of weakened or dead pathogenic cells injected in order to stimulate the production of antibodies 疫苗

ligand /ˈlɪgənd，ˈlaɪ-/ *n*. an atom or molecule or radical or ion that forms a complex around a central atom 配体 配基

eradicate /ɪˈrædɪkeɪt/ *v*. to destroy or get rid of sth completely，especially sth bad 根除；消灭；杜绝

After reading

Task 11   Build your vocabulary. Choose one word which can be used to replace the language shown in bold without changing the meaning of the sentence from the list below. Change forms and cases when necessary.

allege(*v*.)   alter(*v*.)   cease(*v*.)   elaborate(*adj*.)   fragment(*n*.)   philosophy(*n*.)
litigation(*n*.)   induce(*v*.)   reservoir(*n*.)   subside(*v*.)   upsurge(*n*.)

1. They have begun a hunger strike in protest at the **claimed** beating.
   _____

2. In the experiment it was found that in starvation conditions some species **stopped** reproduction and had higher survival rates.
   _____

3. In the case of negative emotions, the functions of communication are fairly straightforward and well **detailed** in the literature.
   _____

4. Fire can drastically **change** forest ecosystems, and this can have important impacts on small mammal abundance, demography and community composition.
   _____

5. They were using genomic tiling microarray, which was constructed with genomic DNA **piece** covering both coding and non-coding sequences.
   _____

6. Every business or organization needs a guiding **thinking** on what they aspire to achieve and what their purpose is.
   _____

7. The result of an economic **increase** should be more land set aside as conservation areas, like wildlife refuges and nature preserves.

8. The Saminists were eventually persecuted, their leaders arrested, and the movement had practically **declined** by 1910, but the idea was planted.
   _____

9. The developing fetal endocrine system can adjust in response to maternally **promoted** changes in its intrauterine environment.
   _____

10. Primary transmission presumably occurs from a **pool** of the pathogen Vibrio cholerae in the aquatic environment.
    _____

Further reading

Baazim, H., Antonio-Herrera, L., Bergthaler, A. (2022). The Interplay of Immunology and Cachexia in Infection and Cancer. *Nature Reviews Immunology*. 22(5).

Croitoru, G. A., et al. (2024). Nanomaterials in Immunology: Bridging Innovative Approaches in Immune Modulation, Diagnostics, and Therapy. *Journal of Functional Biomaterials*. 15(8).

Griffiths, W. J., Wang Y. (2022). Cholesterol Metabolism: from Lipidomics to Immunology. *Journal of Lipid Research*. 63(2).

Tran, H. B., Jakobczak, R., Abdo, A., et al. (2022). Immunolocalization of Zinc Transporters and Metallothioneins Reveals Links to Microvascular Morphology and Functions. *Histochemistry and Cell Biology*. 158(5).

Unit 5
Translational Medicine

Guiding to learn

Translational medicine is a new concept in the field of international biomedical research that appeared in the last 20 years, which transforms basic research into clinical application. Big data and technological innovation have revolutionized medicine and healthcare over the last decade. Translational medicine must be ready to embrace and integrate such tools to augment conventional approaches and nurture new cross-functional collaborations that can maximize the value of data.

Discuss the following questions with your partners.

1. What is gene therapy?
2. What is machine learning?
3. What is translational medicine?

Task 1   Learn the following general academic vocabulary.

feature maintain regulatory transfer consensus considerable criterion initial interaction outcome reliability sequence sufficiently technique code contrast alter external fundamental modification stability domain inhibit neutralization nevertheless transport underlying classical dynamics isolation complementary detection intensive revise anticipate insight mediate

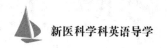

Beginning to read

Task 2   Now read the text.

Translational Medicine: Towards Gene Therapy of Marfan Syndrome
Klaus Kallenbach et al

1. The first descriptions of the Marfan Syndrome（MFS）（马方综合征）by the French paediatrician Antoine Marfan in 1896 and later in the reports of others were based on skeletal features, such as joint contraction, kyphoscoliosis, hypotrophic skeletal muscles(萎缩性骨骼肌), and thin and long extremities, fingers and toes. The American ophthalmologist E. Williams described two families with a luxation of the lenses and other ocular features typical of MFS more than 20 years before Marfan. Today, we know that MFS consists of skeletal, ocular, facial（dysmorphic face）, pulmonary（spontaneous pneumothorax）, dermatologic（striae distensae）, cardiac （mitral valve prolapses）, and, especially, vascular features. The formation of aortic root aneurysms and consecutive acute aortic dissection reduces middle life expectancy （预期寿命）significantly, and MFS is considered a devastating aortic disease.

2. With the development of the Berlin Nosology of Heritable Disorders of Connective Tissue Diseases in 1986, the diagnosis of MFS obtained its first uniformed structure based on clinical features. In early 1990, the FBN1 gene coding for fibrillin was characterized, and it became evident that a mutation in this gene may cause MFS. Therefore, the Berlin nosology was improved and replaced by the stricter Ghent nosology in 1996, where identifying an FBN1 mutation causing MFS was considered a significant criterion for diagnosing MFS. Until now, the revised Ghent nosology, published in 2010, represents the gold standard for diagnosing MFS. FBN1 testing holds much greater weight in the diagnostic assessment now. Next-generation sequencing（NGS）screening of the FBN1 gene and other genes possibly responsible for the hereditary aortic disease（遗传性主动脉疾病）became the standard in the detection of MFS today.

3. Despite the tremendous improvements in understanding the molecular defects underlying MFS and the reliability of the diagnosis, the treatment of MFS has remained almost the same over the last three decades. With the introduction of the prophylactic replacement（预防性替代）of the ascending aorta to avoid the aortic dissection type A in MFS in the late 1970s, the life expectancy of patients with MFS improved from 30—40 years to almost the anticipated average life of the unaffected

population. Certainly, operative standards and techniques improved. Today, a valve-sparing aortic root replacement can be operated with less than 1% operative mortality in specialized centres. New techniques, such as the Personalized External Aortic Root Support (PEARS) (个性化外主动脉根部支架) appeared and arrested attention. In medical drugs, the prophylactic treatment with sartanes may, in combination with beta-blockers, reduce or at least delay the development of the root aneurysm.

4. Other drugs, such as statins, are being investigated based on intensive research and improved molecular biological understanding. Furthermore, the general improvement of the medical armamentarium allows for the enhanced treatment of the ocular and skeletal problems of Marfan patients. Nevertheless, Marfan syndrome remains an incisive illness for the affected patient who fears multiple operations on different organ systems, lifelong medication intake (静脉药物摄入量), reduced opportunities for a regular lifestyle, and possible social isolation.

5. Today, it is general medical knowledge that prophylaxis or even disease avoidance results in a much better outcome than treating the same disorder. Although we can sufficiently diagnose MFS and treat its complications, we cannot cause the illness to disappear. With the concept of translational medicine, we may use the vast amount of knowledge we have collected during the last decades to treat the clinical Marfan syndrome at its root—at the genetic level. With therapeutic gene concepts (治疗性基因概念), it may become possible to alter the genotype of MFS so that the phenotype of the patient appears almost normal without the development of the typical complications.

6. At least two significant obstacles must be overcome before the successful gene therapy of Marfan syndrome becomes a clinical reality. First, the proper genetic target(s) that must be altered need to be identified. Second, a delivery method system that allows permanent expression of the target gene must be developed. We and others have previously discussed different target genes. The TGF-β signalling pathway's pivotal role in developing the MFS vascular phenotype may display potential target genes affecting downstream effector genes, such as Matrix Metalloproteinases (MMPs) (基质金属蛋白酶) and their inhibitors (TIMPs). The transcription factor activator protein－1 (AP－1) (激活蛋白), directly involved in TGF-β signalling and the activation of MMPs, may serve as such a target. We have shown that the neutralization of AP－1 with decoy oligodeoxynucleotides (dODN) (诱骗性寡脱氧核苷酸) technology reduces aortic elastolysis in an established mouse model of MFS. By the modulation of the gene delivery towards RNA hairpin decoy oligonucleotide (dON)-AP1 combined with adeno-associated virus (腺相关病毒) (AAV)-based transduction, we successfully aimed to improve the longevity and stability of AP－1 suppression. Stimulated by these results, we here review our and others' translational gene therapy concepts for Marfan syndrome.

7. Gene therapy opens an exciting new path in managing aortic aneurysm treatment（主动脉瘤治疗）and could，in the long term，be established as a novel option for Marfan syndrome. With the identification of novel therapeutic targets in maintaining endothelial and smooth muscle cell function under stress conditions，recent approaches have been tested in preclinical models. RNA-based therapies have recently gained considerable advances in vascular disease. An overview of targets investigated in preclinical studies is listed in Table 1.

8. One major challenge that limits clinical translation remains the delivery method system. Although adenoviruses proved to have relatively high transduction efficiency in target cells，they are associated with critical safety concerns due to increased inflammation. On the other hand，plasmid-based gene therapy（基因质粒治疗）offers inefficient and transient transduction of targets. In contrast，adeno-associated viruses（AAVs）enable long-term gene expression and represent the most well-studied vector for therapeutic purposes. However，the systemic injection of AAV particles leads to low transduction efficiency in the aortic wall. Local delivery methods based on stents or biocompatible materials（生物相容性材料）have already been established to circumvent these obstacles，improving specificity and efficacy. Additionally，these approaches provide reduced immunogenicity，another major challenge that prevents AAV based strategies from being translated into clinical practice. An extensive summary of the most current delivery methods，modes of application，and possibilities to increase the vascular system's transduction efficiency have been reviewed recently.

9. Studies based on mouse models for Marfan syndrome brought fundamental insights into the molecular mechanisms of the pathophysiology of the disease. However，larger models are essential for further translating pharmacological and gene therapy methods into clinics. Furthermore，small animal models are inefficient for advancing surgical techniques such as local gene delivery. Moreover，due to the similar anatomy to the human subjects，treatments tested in such preclinical studies can be more readily translated into patients. A porcine model for Marfan syndrome based on an FBN1 mutation has been established using genome editing and somatic cell nuclear transfer technologies. The heterozygous animals present classical features described in Marfan patients，such as scoliosis，reduced bone density（骨密度），and the fragmentation of elastic fibres in the aortic wall. Additionally，previous naturally occurring mutations in the fibrillin－1 gene noted in calves brought pathophysiological changes similar to those observed in Marfan patients，including increased aortic dilatation and rupture and mitral valve prolapse and ectopia lenses（屈光不正性角膜透镜）.

10. In conclusion，gene therapy for Marfan syndrome remains a relatively young field. Further studies are required to improve gene transfer to the vascular system in mouse and large animal models.

From Journal of Clinic Medicine，2022，11（14）

New words and expressions

mutation /mjuːˈteɪʃn/ *n*. (genetics) any event that changes genetic structure 突变,变异

prophylaxis /ˌprɒfɪˈlæksɪs/ *n*. the prevention of disease 预防

therapeutic /ˌθerəˈpjuːtɪk/ *adj*. tending to cure or restore to health 治疗的,医疗的

exonuclease /ˌeksəʊˈnjʊklɪˌeɪs/ *n*. a nuclease that releases one nucleotide at a time (serially) beginning at one of a nucleic acid 核酸外切酶

vascular /ˈvæskjələ(r)/ *adj*. of or relating to or having vessels that conduct and circulate fluids 血管的

biocompatible /ˌbaɪəʊkəmˈpætəbl/ *adj*. able to exist together without causing problems 生物相容的,不会引起排斥的

clinical /ˈklɪnɪkl/ *adj*. relating to a clinic or conducted in or as if in a clinic and depending on direct observation of patients 临床的

suppression /səˈpreʃ(ə)n/ *n*. (botany) the failure to develop of some part or organ of a plant 压制,抑制

immunogenicity /ˌɪmjʊnəʊdʒeˈnɪsɪti/ *n*. the ability of a particular substance, such as an antigen or epitope, to provoke an immune response in the body of a human or animal 免疫原性;致免疫力

dilatation /ˌdaɪləˈteʃn/ *n*. the state of being stretched beyond normal dimensions 膨胀,扩张

pivotal /ˈpɪvətl/ *adj*. being of crucial importance 中枢的,重要的

After reading

Task 3 Read Text A again and answer the following questions.

1. How much do you know about Marfan Syndrome (MFS)?

2. What obstacles must be overcome before the gene therapy of Marfan syndrome becomes a clinical reality?

Task 4 Check your vocabulary. Fill in the blanks with the correct form of the words from the following box, each word can be used only once.

aid(*n*.) biology(*n*.) edit(*v*.) enlighten(*v*.) homogeneous(*adj*.) overlap(*v*.)
stress(*n*.) version(*n*.) trait(*n*.) trivial(*adj*.) symptom(*n*.) x-rays(*n*.)

1. Although this may seem _____, the significance of hypobaric environments comes into play when the need to grow plants in space, moons, or planets arises.

2. We found a statistically significant _____ in three of four cases.

3. The most common _____ of COPD is exertional dyspnea that can be accompanied by chronic cough，wheezing，recurrent respiratory infections，fatigue，weight loss, and decreased libido.

4. Future studies may want to use more professional equipment to _____ the video so that the stimuli can be presented longer and larger while still not being consciously visible by participants.

5. Werken provided valuable comments on an earlier _____ of the manuscript.

6. All _____ were taken in the craniocaudal plane.

7. Secondly，once it has been established，it will form dense，_____ stands that will restrict native wetland species from growing in the affected wetland.

8. More and more studies are currently underway investigating the effects of an externally applied electric field to a cell's _____.

9. It was shown that body color and eye color are linked on chromosome two，and that the wing venation _____ was present on chromosome three.

10. There are of course many concerns with possession by malevolent entities，but also various trends of being possessed by beneficial spirits or benevolent space aliens come to _____ primitive earth people.

Task 5 Build your vocabulary. Read the sentences below, and decide which word in each bracket is more suitable.

1. Healthy rivers will be able to （soak up/absorb） a fair amount of nutrients and bacteria before the oxygen levels drop to dangerous levels.

2. ER homeostasis apparatus reduces BTZ lethality，（contrary/unlike） to expectation.

3. R.norvegicus likes to live close to the ground，and is also not as adaptable，making it easier to （expel/suspend） or exterminate from buildings.

4. There are several （groups/categories） of tannins that are found in plants，but condensed tannins are the form commonly found in aspen.

5. It is the recommendation the government needs to make and to help Americans （implement/start） in their lifestyles if there is any hope or reversing the current cycle of obesity and disease.

6. Here，it could be concluded that a clear （honest/objective） and sufficient evidence of the underlying hazard or disadvantages play a vital role in attracting people to take part in a social movement.

7. Any interested actor can attempt to influence MMS's and Alaska's decisions although the agencies will have little reason to （answer/respond） unless a significant majority of locals are against leasing.

8. This information will give insight into when the necessary genes are activated or repressed，and the （duration/time） of the gene activity will reflect its importance in the stressful situation.

9. All measurements were square-root (modified/transformed) to improve normality.

10. Most COCs do not completely (stop/suppress) ovarian follicular development.

Guiding to learn

Task 6 Learn the following general academic vocabulary.

available constitute identification individual principle sector source variability complex computational consequently evaluation feature participatory regulatory relevance strategic commentary component core demonstrate framework illustrate initially interaction maximize registration sequential validation attribute dimension emerge hypothesis integrate multidimensional output alteration fundamental generation medical perspective sustaine accuracy diverse enhance inhibition initiate intelligence transform underlying unprecedented dynamic innovation paradigm prioritize reverse simulate ultimately unique automation crucial highlight random reinforcement thereby virtual accommodate revolutionize assemble

Beginning to read

Task 7 Now read the text.

Text B

Application of Machine Learning in Translational Medicine: Current Status and Future Opportunities

Nadia Terranova et al

1. Big data and technological innovation have revolutionized medicine and healthcare over the last decade. Today, advanced technological solutions are able to generate health and medical data at the individual level in real time and in a real-world environment. They are at the core of such digital disruption that holds promise for improving the practice of medicine towards a more targeted and personalized paradigm, enabled by data-driven decisions based on real-world evidence, patient-

participatory（患者参与性）drug development，and healthcare democratization. In recent years，pharmaceutical Research and Development（R&D）has transformed to a highly dynamic process enabled by patient-centered iterative forward and reverse translation. Traversing the path from idea to medicine has become increasingly multidisciplinary and inter-connected，as exemplified by the Drug Discovery，Development，and Deployment Map，illustrating a network view of the process and associated cross-sector ecosystem，challenging the typical chevron（linear，sequential，left to right）view of pharmaceutical R&D pipeline . A Bayesian learning mindset that exploits the totality of evidence is particularly important in timely delivery of innovative healthcare solutions to address unmet medical needs with the right sense of urgency.

2. Whereas advances in biology，biomedical engineering，and computational sciences have resulted in an explosive increase in our ability to generate and store multidimensional data from diverse sources，consistent real-time integration of these data for principled and timely decision making in pharmaceutical R&D and healthcare remains aspirational. Recognizing this critical importance of optimal knowledge management，the pharmaceutical industry has started building digital capabilities and embracing innovations in Data Science into their Research and Development（R&D）organizations. Machine learning（ML），deep learning（DL）and more generally artificial intelligence（AI）techniques are central components of this innovation. While AI refers to the output of a computer generated by mimicking a human behavior（模仿人类行为）and it does not say how the problem has been solved，ML is a subset of AI consisting of a set of algorithms that parse data，learn from them，and then apply learnings to make intelligent decisions. A simple and widely used classification of ML algorithms is into supervised，unsupervised，DL and then reinforcement learning. Supervised learning is task driven and it is used for classification and prediction tasks on new data by starting on datasets with known labels or outcomes. Differently，unsupervised learning methods are data driven and focus on finding structures and patterns inside the data itself. Examples include finding groups and clusters（clustering），understanding relationships between items（association rule mining），and finding a more compact representation of the data（dimension reduction）. Reinforcement learning uses algorithms interactively learning to react to an environment from mistakes by focusing on decision and policy making. Lastly，inspired by the biological neural network（NN）（神经网络）of the human brain，DL uses NNs with many layers to solve the hardest（for computers）problems. Such process of learning is far more capable than that of standard ML models. Indeed，while both ML and DL fall under the broad category of AI，DL is what powers the most human-like artificial intelligence（类人的人工智能）.

3. Owing to their ability to learn hidden and predictive patterns in large amounts of heterogenous（大量异质性）and high-dimensional datasets（高维数据集），AI

techniques have been increasingly adopted across the drug discovery and development value chain. Initially, AI methods were mostly used in drug discovery to analyze large sets of chemical structure data, gene expression and genetic data, and high throughput in vitro data. Optimization of drug candidates towards better drug properties has been an area of sustained focus of AI/ML frameworks in drug discovery, enabling efficient iterative approaches to multi-dimensional optimization based on virtual screening and prediction of physicochemical properties and biological activity and toxicity. More recently, a wide range of ML applications have emerged as promising approaches to generate new knowledge in translational and clinical drug development. Together with the automation of process pipelines and operational design, the integration and analysis of large, multi-dimensional, and heterogenous data sets, such as-omics data, information from wearable devices, images, and electronic health records, offers an unprecedented opportunity for AI/ML applications in drug development. The associated contexts of use range broadly from advancing understanding of the disease and its underlying physiological and biological underpinnings, elucidation of drug mechanism of action（MoA）（药物作用机理）and identification of promising combinations, characterization of sources of population variability in patients' response, and enhancement of trial design and operational efficiency, diagnosis, individualized treatment, and precision dosing solutions .

4. The integration and use of AI/ML methods across the translational through clinical drug development continuum have already demonstrated a clear impact on our ability to successfully maximize the value of data. Furthermore, these methods have enhanced knowledge management both with respect to the studied drug and the disease/patient population, thereby enabling optimization of R&D across the three key inter-dependent strategic pillars that constitute the practice of Translational Medicine: target, patient, and dose. These pillars represent the fundamental pivots for hypothesis generation and ultimately for data-driven knowledge generation from preclinical, clinical, and regulatory evaluations designed to build a body of scientific evidence to achieve clinical proof of concept of innovative investigational therapies. Robust and efficient data-driven optimization alongside these three pillars is crucial to maximize probability of success in clinical development and ultimately to successfully impact product registration, labeling, and guidance for therapeutic use at the right dosage and in the context of applicable personalized medicine strategies in concert with companion diagnostics（伴生诊断）where relevant, to maximize benefit/risk across populations and clinical contexts of use. A quantitative mindset that collaboratively synergizes the disciplines of biomarker sciences, pharmacometrics, systems pharmacology, and bioinformatics is vitally important to the successful practice of Translational Medicine. Accordingly, advanced analytics represents a key enabler for Translational Medicine to innovatively support forward and reverse translation（逆

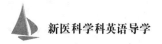
转录）.

5. In this commentary, we provide an overview of ML applications in drug discovery and development, aligned with the three strategic pillars of Translational Medicine and offer perspectives on their potential to transform the science and practice of the discipline.

6. The objective of the "target" strategic pillar is to identify the right biological target for a selected disease. Confidence in the biological target and therapeutic hypothesis must be built to initiate the discovery of drugs modulating this target and consequently the disease. This process, also known as target selection and validation, is data driven. It uses a wide range of experiments and multi-dimensional datasets that can inform the identification and selection of novel targets and provide evidence of their association with a disease. Various ML applications using computational druggability prediction methods（计算药物预测方法）have emerged for prioritizing target selection by reducing the potential space of druggable targets, and for elucidating the target-disease（疾病靶向）causality. These include the prediction of druggable genes at the genome-wide scale by constructing, for example, a decision tree-based meta-classifier and training it on data including network topological features, tissue expression profile, and subcellular localization. Use cases accommodate predictions for specific cancer types based on a variety of genomic and systemic datasets fed into a support vector machine（SVM）（支持向量机）classifier and then target validation through inhibition with antibodies, synthetic peptides, and small molecules. Supervised ML classifiers predicting whether a small-molecule drug can be generated for any given target have also been generated by integrating rich data including physicochemical, structural, and geometric attributes. Emerging and novel therapeutic modalities will demand unique considerations. Of relevance for improved patient stratification, Iorio et al. identified oncogenic alterations in tumors and found associations with drug sensitivity/resistance, thus highlighting the importance of tissue lineage in mediating drug response .Significant work has been done for designing and screening effective drug combinations which are commonly used to treat patients with complex diseases that respond poorly to single-agent therapies. For example, a novel network propagation-based method with Random Forest（RF）（随机森林）models predicting anticancer drug synergy to the accuracy of experimental replicates has been established by integrating the cross-cell and cross-drug information from a large drug combination screening dataset and assembling the information in monotherapy and simulated molecular data. Recent advances in natural language processing（NLP）have further unlocked information and knowledge on targets and target-disease association present in literature data by enabling effective and efficient access to available and unstructured sources. These methods can additionally be deployed for elucidating the molecular basis of drug-related toxicities（药物相关毒性）resulting from off-target

interactions，thereby informing hypothesis generation for next-generation（"best-in-class"）drug design aimed at maximizing therapeutic index.

7. A key component in target validation is building of confidence in the therapeutic hypothesis using quantitative systems pharmacology（QSP）（定量系统药理学）models. Such mechanistic models integrate information on drug pharmacokinetics（PK）[药物（代谢）动力学]，target binding，and biological processes of interest and mechanisms of action，resulting from prior knowledge and available preclinical and clinical data，to quantitatively predict efficacy and safety responses over time and translate molecular data to clinical outcomes. QSP provides an ideal quantitative framework for integration of diverse big data sources，including omics and imaging，the dimensionality of which can be reduced by using ML methods. By allowing the identification of relevant association and data representations，the development of QSP platforms with higher granularity and enhanced predictive power can be further enhanced.

From The AAPS Journal，*2021*，*23*（*74*）

After reading

Task 8　Build your vocabulary.

Directions：Match the following words with their corresponding definitions and Chinese equivalents.

English：accommodate　access　attribute　components　dimension　framework　hypothesis　integrate　innovation　initiate　intelligent　mechanism　paradigm　perspective　registration

Chinese：适应　接触（权）　特征　成分　范围　结构　假说　整合　创新　开始　智能　的　机制　范例　看法　注册

Paras. 1—7

English	Chinese	Definition
1. _____	_____	a. the act of starting something for the first time; introducing something new
2. _____	_____	b. a standard or typical example
3. _____	_____	c. magnitude or extent
4. _____	_____	d. having the capacity for thought and reason especially to a high degree

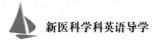

5. _____   _____   e. the underlying structure

6. _____   _____   f. a construct whereby objects or individuals can be distinguished

7. _____   _____   g. make into a whole or make part of a whole

8. _____   _____   h. the act of enrolling

9. _____   _____   i. a tentative theory about the natural world; a concept that is not yet verified but that if true would explain certain facts or phenomena

10. _____   _____   j. a way of regarding situations or topics etc

11. _____   _____   k. bring into being

12. _____   _____   l. make fit for, or change to suit a new purpose

13. _____   _____   m. the right to obtain or make use of or take advantage of something

14. _____   _____   n. an abstract part of something

15. _____   _____   o. the philosophical theory that all phenomena can be explained in terms of physical or biological causes

Guiding to learn

Task 9   Learn the following general academic vocabulary from the word bank.

> distinctive persist abnormal eliminate dominant internalized evolution
> mediate conversely maintenance negatively impact induce consistent
> demonstrate release distinct nevertheless contrast undergo involvement
> diverse

Beginning to read

Task 10   Now read the text.

Text C

Cell-in-Cell: From Cell Biology to Translational Medicine
Qiao Chen et al

1. Cell-in-cell structures (CICs)(细胞内结构), characterized by one or more live cells (referred to as effector cells) internalized into another cells, have been considered simple physiological or pathological phenomena without extensive biological significance. For decades, researchers mainly emphasized morphological descriptions and observed CICs by microscopy in a wide range of cell types and tissues, both in vivo and in vitro. In general, CICs commonly occur at a rate of 0.3%—2.5% of the total sample population in a wide range of carcinomas, while surprisingly, in some cases, CIC formation is as high as ~6% in heterogeneous breast cancer tissue in a patient with poor prognosis . Currently, CICs are attracting increasing attention because of their correlation with various physiological and pathological conditions, their involvement in inflammation and carcinoma initiation and progression, and their potential implications in translational medicine. CICs occur universally in diverse tissues; therefore, establishing how the functional status of CICs influences diseases and treatment response is important. Efforts to explore the clinic-pathological (临床病理的)correlates of CICs in patients will provide new approaches to disease treatment and prevention. For the purposes of discussion, CICs will be divided into two basic types: homotypic CICs, in which both of the effector and host cells are the same cell type, and heterotypic CICs, in which the effector cell is internalized into a host of a different cell type. Notably, important breakthroughs have been made the possible mechanisms and potential significance of CICs, including homotypic CICs, referred to as entosis, and heterotypic CICs, referred to emperipolesis(伸入运动), which have clinical and potential therapeutic applications.

2. The molecular mechanisms and core elements underlying the formation of homotypic CICs has been reviewed recently. Homotypic CIC formation is induced in response to any of the following stimuli: low energy states by glucose withdrawal, aberrant shape regulation of invading cells in mitosis, and detachment of effector cells

from the extracellular matrix（细胞外基质）. Subsequently，CIC invasion is regulated genetically by three core machineries，including intact adherens junctions（AJs）（粘附连接），imbalance of contractile actomyosin（CA）（收缩肌动球蛋白）of invading cells，and the mechanical ring（MR）between the peripheries of invading and engulfing cells. Cells activated the phosphorylation of myosin light chain（MLC2）（肌球蛋白轻链）and diaphanous-related formin1（mDia1）with higher RhoA activity，thereby producing biophysical forces that drive penetration，representing an intriguing and distinctive form of phagocytosis. At the interface between the two cells，E-cadherin-mediated AJs interact with F-actin through α-catenin，β-catenin，and vinculin and form a ring-like structure termed the mechanical ring，which is involved in homotypic CIC formation.

3. Following entry into the cytoplasm of the host cell，there are several possible fates for the internalized cell. It might persist as a live cell and even undergo cell division while still internalized. However，the most common fate for the internalized cells is lysosomal cell death（溶酶体细胞死亡）. Recently，Overholtzer et al. defined a nonapoptotice cell death program mediated by CIC process，entosis，in which suspended epithelial cells actively invasive and the cells die inside their neighboring host cell. Entosis is involved in the linker cell clearance in Caenorhabditis elegans（秀丽隐杆线虫）and in luminal epithelial cell（腔内上皮细胞）elimination in embryo implantation，suggesting that entosis is an ancient process to regulate key events required for embryonic development. Entosis occurs from bacteria to mammals，it indicates that entotic process is conserved across evolution. Consistent with this model，entosis contributes to cell competition in Drosophila by controlling the process by which "fit" cells eliminate their less fit neighbors and can also mediate cell completion in tumor cells Cell competition mediated by entosis plays both promotive and suppressive roles in tumors. "Winner" cells（hosts）use entosis as a mechanism of cell competition to kill "loser" cells（engulfed cells）（吞噬细胞）and become clonally dominant in a heterogeneous population，suggesting that entosis for cell competition contributes to clonal selection in tumor evolution. Moreover，nutrients，such as amino acid and glucose，are provided following engulfed cell death and degradation，which promotes the survival of the host cell under starvation conditions. Strikingly，host cells not only benefit from the nutrients released by the engulfed cells but also experience multinucleation because of the steric interference by the engulfed cells，propagating genomic instability and thereby driving tumor progression. In addition，host cells with mutated p53 often survive following abnormal mitotic events，which indicates that mutated p53 is associated with CIC's contribution to genomic instability for tumor progression. Nevertheless，entosis inhibits tumorigenesis by eliminating cells detached from the extracellular matrix. Further research supports this view that host cells engulf cells with aberrant mitosis as a tumorsuppressive act of "assisted suicide"（协助自杀），indicating entosis as an antitumorigenic effect in cancer. A recent study indicated that

in a nontumor context，aneuploid daughter cells（非整倍体子细胞）during the entotic process are engulfed and eliminated by host cells，thus playing a surveillance role in the maintenance of genome integrity. Therefore，identifying and characterizing the mechanisms of entosis in different cellular and molecular contexts would be helpful to further understand its biological effects in physiological and pathological processes.

From BioMed Research International，2022（1）：7608521

New words and expressions

glucose /ˈgluːkəʊs/ *n*. a monosaccharide sugar that has several forms 葡萄糖

carcinoma /ˌkɑːsɪˈnəʊmə/ *n*. a cancer that affects the top layer of the skin or the lining of the organs inside the stomach 癌（影响上皮组织或腹腔器官内膜的恶性肿瘤）

detachment /dɪˈtætʃmənt/ *n*. the act of releasing from an attachment or connection 分离

intact /ɪnˈtækt/ *adj*. complete and not damaged 未受损伤的，完好无损

cytoplasm /ˈsaɪtəʊplæzəm/ *n*. the protoplasm of a cell excluding the nucleus 细胞质

penetration /ˌpenɪˈtreʃ(ə)n/ *n*. the act of entering into or through something 渗透；穿刺

embryonic /ˌembrɪˈɑnɪk/ *adj*. of an organism prior to birth or hatching 胚胎的

metastatic /ˌmetəˈstætɪk/ *n*. the spreading of a disease to another part of the body 转移

surveillance /sɜːˈveɪləns/ *n*. close observation of a person or group 监视；监控

implantation /ˌɪmplɑːnˈteʃən/ *n*. a surgical procedure that places something in the human body 植入

mammal /ˈmæml/ *n*. young are born alive except for the small subclass of monotremes and nourished with milk 哺乳动物

internalize /ɪnˈtɜːnəlaɪz/ *v*. incorporate within oneself 使内在化

After reading

Task 11   **Build your vocabulary. Choose one word which can be used to replace the language shown in bold without changing the meaning of the sentence from the list below. Change forms and cases when necessary.**

advocate contract compound dictate graph insisted preliminary retard subtle tiny transferred

1. In many other countries national regulations **lay down** the terms of egg donation.

_____

2. Thimerosal is an organomercurial **combination** composed of 50% mercury by weight in the form of ethylmercury that is bound to thiosalicylate. _____

3. The progression of the disease can be **delayed** by early surgery. _____

4. The White women coders may have not detected **slight** differences in ethinic/ cultural responses and expressions.

5. Nurse leaders **support** for the use of standardized nursing terminologies in electronic records.

6. **Initial** verbal evaluations from the school nurse and a few students have been positive. _____

7. The Pitocin running was increased in order to **shrink** the uterus and prevent hemorrhaging. _____

8. It is simply amazing just how much this **very small** wing in a giant hospital does to treat spinal cord injuries and just how much I have become a part of it in just a few weeks of volunteering. _____

9. Under the current system, she was unable to stay at UMHS as an involuntary patient and was thus **relocated** to another institution. _____

10. Below is a **chart** of concentrations and time distribution of plasma nicotine in various nicotine substances. _____

Further reading

Chen Q, Wang X, He M.(2022). Cell-in-Cell: From Cell Biology to Translational Medicine. *BioMed Research International*. Sep 14.

Fosse, V., Oldoni, E., Gerardi, C., et al. (2022). Evaluating Translational Methods for Personalized Medicine-A Scoping Review. *Journal of Personalized Medicine*. 12(7).

Kallenbach, K., Remes, A., Müller, O. J., et al. (2022). Translational Medicine: Towards Gene Therapy of Marfan Syndrome. *Journal of Clinic Medicine*. 11(14).

Schulte, P. A., Guerin, R. J., Cunningham, T. R., et al. (2022). Applying Translational Science Approaches to Protect Workers Exposed to Nanomaterials. *Front Public Health*. Jun 10.

Terranova, N., Venkatakrishnan, K., Benincosa, L. J. (2022). Application of Machine Learning in Translational Medicine: Current Status and Future Opportunities. *The AAPS Journal*. 23(4).

Unit 6
Translational Therapeutics

Guiding to learn

Ischemic stroke and traumatic brain injury (TBI) are among the leading causes of death and disability worldwide with impairments ranging from mild to severe. Neurotrophic factors such as brain-derived neurotrophic factor (BDNF) and nerve growth factor (NGF) serve as potential therapeutic options to increase neural repair and recovery as they promote neuroprotection and regeneration. Non-infectious intestinal disease is a major cause of morbidity and mortality. To improve treatment of intestinal disease, large animal models are increasingly recognized as critical tools to translate the basic science discoveries made in rodent models into clinical application. Neuronal microcircuits in psychology, physiology, pharmacology and pathology make the neuronal ensembles theoretical framework a dynamic neuroscience paradigm.

Discuss the following questions with your partners.

1. What are the challenges in translating these brain-derived neurotrophic factor and nerve growth factor therapeutics from the bench to the clinic?
2. Why are pigs used as model of enteric diseases?
3. How much do you know about neuronal ensembles from synaptic to functional connectivity?

Task 1   Learn the following general academic vocabulary.

available distribution administration appropriate impact regulate selective compensate consensus contribute demonstrate outcome reactive validation compounded modify incorporate inhibit reveal underlie utility comprehensive elimination intervention induce minimize restoration route sphere trigger

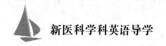

Beginning to read

Task 2   Now read the text.

Text A

Brain-Derived Neurotrophic Factor and Nerve Growth Factor Therapeutics for Brain Injury: The Current Translational Challenges in Preclinical and Clinical Research

Serena-Kaye Sims et al

1. Ischemic stroke(缺血性中风), a leading cause of disability worldwide, results from limited blood flow to the brain due to the block-age or narrowing of arteries. Unfortunately, there are a lack of therapeutic options that can effectively minimize damage or aid in recovery following brain injury from ischemic stroke. The pharmacologic standard of care involves clot breakdown with the thrombolytic agent tissue plasminogen activator (tPA)(组织型纤溶酶原激活物) and/or prevention of further ischemia using anticoagulants such as aspirin. After a stroke, tPA is often the best available option for patients but must be administered within the first 3 hours, or potentially up to 4.5 hours. The short time window in which tPA can be administered, combined with potential complications such as intracranial hemorrhage, has greatly limited its use in some patients. While clot thrombolysis and prevention can be useful in preventing further ischemic damage, by the time a stroke patient receives these treatments, brain injury has already occurred. Despite a need for new stroke treatments, there has been little success in identifying therapeutics that can be widely used to promote neural repair and improve functional recovery following brain injury. Many promising experimental treatments have failed to deliver positive results in clinical trials for reasons including lack of efficacy and target validation and pharmacokinetic and pharmacodynamic issues.

2. One avenue of stroke research has involved exploring the use of neurotrophin treatments(神经营养因子治疗) as a mechanism for neural repair and enhanced recovery. Neurotrophins are a family of growth factors that play important roles in the survival and function of neurons. There are four known members of the neurotrophin family of growth factors in mammals: brain-derived neurotrophic factor (BDNF)(脑源性神经营养因子), nerve growth factor (NGF), neurotrophin-3 (NT-3), and neurotrophin 4 (NT-4). Neurotrophins regulate development in the central and

peripheral nervous systems by interacting with tropomyosin receptor kinase（Trk）（原肌球蛋白受体激酶）receptors. NGF preferentially binds with TrkA receptors，BDNF and NT－4 with TrkB receptors，and NT－3 with TrkC receptors. The dimerization and autophosphorylation of Trk receptors activate major signaling pathways including PLC-gamma，MAPK/ERK，and PI3K/Akt which suppress apoptosis through their downstream mediators CREB，BCL2，and BAX and Bad，respectively. BDNF and NGF increase the phosphorylation of synapsin 1 for synaptic vesicle release. These four neurotrophins also bind to their low-affinity receptor，p75NTR，which induces apoptosis，and in some cases may promote neuronal survival and neurite growth during neurodevelopment. Therefore，neurotrophins are key mediators in neural plasticity postinjury to promote neuronal growth and survival. Of these four neurotrophins，only two，BDNF and NGF，are well studied as potential stroke treatments.

3. This review will outline the current state of preclinical and clinical research surrounding the potential for BDNF and NGF to become treatment options for patients following stroke. These neurotrophins promote neuroprotection and regeneration and have been examined to determine their role in neural repair as well as their ability to improve functional recovery in preclinical and，to a lesser extent，clinical studies. Direct and indirect methods of increasing levels of these neurotrophins in animal models have demonstrated promise in improving outcome measures following brain injury. Unfortunately，the translation of these preclinical studies into clinical trials has been limited. This review will focus on both direct administration of exogenous neurotrophic factors（外源性神经营养因子） and indirect methods of modifying endogenous neurotrophic factor levels in the central nervous system after stroke，and it will also examine the challenges involved in moving BDNF and NGF-related treatments from the bench to the clinic.

4. *Challenges with Treatments*. Currently，a need exists for the development of additional therapies that are effective for improving recovery from ischemic injury. While there have been promising advances in preclinical studies，many of these therapies have failed to translate clinically. There are several challenges that may contribute to this lack of translation. First，many treatments have poor pharmacokinetic profiles. Second，the presence of the blood-brain barrier limits the ability of many systemically administered therapeutics to access the central nervous system. Finally，preclinical studies vary widely in their methods，and their outcomes have not converged on a consensus as to the effects of neurotrophin treatment or the extent of those effects. These issues may contribute to the challenges in translating preclinical studies into clinical trials. Human trials involving the administration of neurotrophins for ischemic injury（缺血性损伤） are rare，and there have been no large，comprehensive clinical trials. As a result，there is not sufficient information to assess whether current preclinical models and methodologies are adequate to forecast human

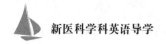

outcomes.

5. *Poor Pharmacokinetics*. Neurotrophins can form protein-antibody（蛋白质抗体）complexes which may affect their tissue distribution, metabolism, and elimination. Additionally, peptidases and proteases in the blood can degrade neurotrophins, leading to reduced bioavailability, as evidenced by poor tissue distribution and short half-lives. An increased dose would be required to compensate for its poor bioavailability. This, in turn, can trigger adverse effects. Administration of neurotrophins can cause immunogenicity which can manifest in adverse effects including hypersensitivity and anaphylactic shock. In order to overcome these pharmacokinetic issues, neurotrophins have been incorporated in drug delivery systems and neurotrophin mimetics（神经营养因模拟）with more favorable pharmacokinetics have been developed. Studies involving the implantation of BDNF polymers in the hippocampi of rats indicated that microspheres released the majority of the encapsulated BDNF within 48 hours. Mimetics, which mimic the BDNF protein, were similarly created in an attempt to circumvent the pharmacokinetic issues. The development of nonpeptide molecules that can activate the TrkB receptor without activating the harmful p75NTR receptor has been the subject of current research. In vitro experiments demonstrate that the molecule LM22A-4, a selective small-molecule partial agonist of TrkB, can trigger the downstream activators of the TrkB receptor. Although these interventions are still in the preclinical stage, their potential to overcome pharmacokinetic challenges may lead to future use in clinical trials.

6. *Poor Blood-Brain Barrier Permeability*. Attempts to use BDNF and NGF as therapeutics for central nervous system（CNS）disorders typically utilize central administration routes that bypass the BBB, including intra-cerebroventricular（ICV）（脑室内的）injection, intraparenchymal（器官实质内的）injection, and intranasal administration. This is largely due to their severe limitation in crossing the blood-brain barrier; however, challenges related to direct central administration still remain. Intracerebroventricular and intraparenchymal routes of administration are highly invasive. Although intranasal administration is noninvasive, it generally results in lower efficiency of drug delivery to brain tissues as nasal mucosa can inhibit molecule permeability which is compounded by a lack of literature on appropriate nasal delivery. The lack of methods for efficient and noninvasive delivery of BDNF and NGF to the brain has therefore presented a road-block to studying the direct administration of these neurotrophins.

7. Indirect modification is achieved by the administration of therapeutics that elicit an increase in neurotrophins in the CNS, including drugs classified as NMDA receptor antagonists, cholinesterase inhibitors, statins, and sigma-1 receptor agonists. NMDA receptor antagonists, including memantine（美金刚）, ketamine, and dextromethorphan, have been used in humans as experimental therapeutics for stroke.

NMDA receptor antagonism is a mechanism of action in several Alzheimer's disease therapeutics(阿尔茨海默病治疗)，including memantine. In addition to NMDA receptor antagonism，memantine was found to increase BDNF levels in macaques，as measured by upregulated mRNA and protein expression of BDNF. Because of this impact on neurotrophic factor expression，memantine and other NMDA receptor antagonists are being studied as potential stroke therapeutics in animal models as well as in human clinical trials. One completed trial investigating memantine as a therapeutic for poststroke aphasia showed that memantine treatment resulted in an improvement in speech compared to placebo but did not measure BDNF levels，so it is unclear what mechanisms underlie the benefits to speech associated with memantine treatment. In mice，memantine resulted in increased BDNF signaling，a reduction in reactive astrogliosis(活性星形胶质细胞增生)，improved vascularization，and improvements in functional recovery. In addition to memantine，several other therapeutics have been shown to modify BDNF levels. Donepezil，a cholinesterase inhibitor used for the treatment of Alzheimer's disease，increased serum BDNF in Alzheimer's disease patients，while atorvastatin，a HMG-CoA reductase inhibitor，increased serum BDNF levels and improved functional recovery following stroke.

8. Stem cell therapy is another method currently being studied for its potential to increase BDNF levels. In vitro studies have shown that neural progenitor cells are capable of releasing neurotrophins including BDNF，NGF，and NT－3. Further preclinical studies have demonstrated the utility of stem cells to elevate BDNF in models of neurological disorders. Implantation of neural stem cells yielded elevated BDNF and increased synaptic density(突触密度) in a mouse model of Alzheimer's disease while mouse models of ischemia reveal that administration of embryonic stem cells (ESCs) can lead to the restoration of behavioral deficits，synaptic connections，and damaged neurons through the release of neurotrophic factors such as BDNF，NGF，and GDNF.

From Neural Plasticity，*2022(1)：3889300*

New words and expressions

pharmacologic /ˌfɑːməkəˈlɒdʒɪk/ *adj*. of or relating to pharmacology 药理学的，药物学的

thrombolytic /ˌθrɒmbəʊˈlɪtɪk/ *n*. a kind of pharmaceutical that can break up clots blocking the flow of blood to the heart muscle 溶血栓药

ischemia /ˈɪskiːmɪə/ *n*. local anemia in a given body part sometimes resulting from vasoconstriction or thrombosis or embolism 局部缺血

hemorrhage /ˈhemərɪdʒ/ *n*. flow of blood from a ruptured blood vessels 出血

avenue /ˈævənjuː/ *n*. a choice or way of making progress towards sth 方式，方法，途径

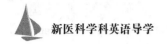
downstream /ˌdaʊnˈstriːm/ *adv*. in the direction in which a river flows 顺流而下；在下游方向

hypersensitivity /ˌhaɪpəˌsensəˈtɪvəti/ *n*. extreme sensitivity 超敏反应；过敏性

encapsulate /ɪnˈkæpsjʊleɪt/ *vt*. to express the most important parts of sth in a few words，a small space or a single object 简述；概括；压缩；封装；形成胶囊

preclinical /priːˈklɪnɪk(ə)l/ *adj*. of or relating to the early phases of a disease when accurate diagnosis is not possible because symptoms of the disease have not yet appeared 临床前的

After reading

Task 3   Read Text A again and answer the following questions.

1. How much do you know about brain-derived neurotrophic factor and nerve growth factor therapeutics?

2. What's the meaning of indirect modifiction?

Task 4   Check your vocabulary. Fill in the blanks with the correct form of the words from the following box, each word can be used only once.

academic(*adj*.)	arouse (*v*.)	benefit (*n*.)	compute (*v*.)	contend (*v*.)
degenerate(*adj*.)	hierarchy(*n*.)	instinct(*n*.)	interlocking(*adj*.)	metabolism(*n*.)
radical(*adj*.)	strata(*n*.)			

1. Investing in computers for our schools would make it possible for teachers to use these and other content specific programs to improve motivation and _____ success in all students.

2. If the desiccation response isn't necessary for adaptation to low pressure，and really is a side effect of the plant perceiving low pressures as lower humidity，then the induction of the pathways is causing a drain on _____.

3. With the inherent bias of the health care system within the socioeconomic _____ regarding access to contraceptives，there come implications of who should and should not be bearing children.

4. While she was filling out paperwork in the emergency department，staff noticed she began to have trouble keeping her eyes open. Her vital signs were taken and were stable and she was easily _____.

5. Yet，regardless of the long litany of potential reasons why the decrease in HIV vertical transfer has been sluggish in its descent one of the larges reasons for the possible failure is due to the _____ societal constrains that negatively impact a woman even before MTCT.

6. Despite the problems associated with sample size, the results indicated that reproduction is high on the _____ of biological functions.

7. Women who do not choose to terminate unplanned pregnancies will require costly pre-and post-natal care, and will undergo _____ bodily changes that could endanger their health.

8. To address the first hypothesis, planned contrasts (ANOVA) were conducted to _____ BP changes from Time 1 to Time 2, and again at the end of the study.

9. However, the _____ of such projects aren't always clear even upon completion.

10. Secondly, the energy levels are massively _____.

Task 5 Read the sentences below, decide which word in each bracket more suitable.

1. In this process, participants held meetings and set goals at the very beginning of the collective (protest/complaint).

2. However, it is not clear whether these two proteins (interact/cooperate) through direct binding, if they form a complex that binds DNA and whether sox17 promoter is one of their shared target.

3. In contrast, for rainfall, a (medium-size/middle-sized) cluster (districts number 4, 5, 11 and 14) of low values appears in the central northern region.

4. In this case, citizens become wary of the plant after an (abnormal/unlikely) and particularly devastating amount of birth defects were occurring among newborns in their small community.

5. Community members who (participated/contributed) in the design of the greenway showed long term commitment and stewardship to the area's public building and green spaces.

6. Bell does say that the facts of physics do not (oblige/force) us to accept one philosophy rather than the other.

7. The uptake of water by glaciers would have lowered sea level as well. For tetrapods living in coastal habitats, these compounding factors would have led to a great (decline/decrease) in available habitat.

8. For African American women, communication is more than mere words. Emotions as expressed by the speaker's (tone /style) are indicative of the person's beliefs.

9. For the issue of change concerning circumcision, a person may decide to (commit/perform) to their prior knowledge of the procedure during any point of the process.

10. Their focus was primarily on the use of the computer system to improve the quality of nursing documentation as measured by the Joint Commission on Accreditation of Healthcare Organizations (JCAHO), rather than on the (vocabulary/terminology) used to document nursing care.

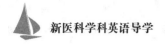

Guiding to learn

Task 6   Learn the following general academic vocabulary.

constitute define distribution variation complexity evaluate feature maintenance
regulator contribute criteria demonstrate layer sequence sufficient validate
attribute contrast overall projection subsequent summarize compound generate
modify ratio aggregate discriminate inhibit initiate transport utilize comprise
innovation intervention release ultimately appendix induce restore

Beginning to read

Task 7   Now read the text.

 Text B

Use of Translational, Genetically Modified Porcine Models to Ultimately Improve Intestinal Disease Treatment

Cecilia R. Schaaf and Liara M. Gonzalez

1. Gastrointestinal disease（肠胃疾病） accounts for over 3.0 million hospitalizations and over ＄135.9 billion in health care expenditures per year. To lessen this incredible burden to patients and our healthcare system，animal models play a critical role in discovery of intestinal disease pathogenesis and therapeutic innovation. For successful clinical translation，it is critical that animal models are properly validated. The criteria used to validate an animal model include certifying similarity in biology and clinical presentation between model and human disease（face validity）， confirming that clinical interventions（临床干预）produce similar effects（predictive ability），and demonstrating that the target under investigation has a similar role in the model compared to human clinical disease（target validity）. Of intestinal disease animal models，rodents are historically preferred for use due to their low cost and maintenance，rapid reproduction，and readily available rodent-specific reagents. However，it is now widely recognized that rodents do not fully mimic human disease，

physiology, immunology, or drug metabolism(药物代谢), thus limiting their use as pre-clinical models for disease treatment. For example, despite promising pre-clinical murine anti-cancer therapeutic studies, success rate of these therapeutics in human clinical trial is only around 5%. Furthermore, the small size of rodents makes it difficult to model and advance surgical and endoscopic techniques. The differences between rodents and humans have left gaps in both basic science research and pre-clinical model development for intestinal diseases.

2. To better represent both human physiology and disease, and aid in the discovery of new treatments, porcine models are gaining popularity. With similar genome, size and architecture of the intestine, omnivorous diet, microbiome, immunology, and physiology to humans, pigs are increasingly the preferred model of enteric diseases (Table 1). The large size of the pig allows for multiple, longitudinal sampling from the same individual. Their large litter size of around 12 piglets allows for ease of gender and sibling matching. These attributes reduce both experimental variation as well as overall animal use. Additionally, for toxicology and drug discovery testing, pigs have oral and parenteral dosing rates similar to humans as well as similar responses to a variety of drug classes.

3. Grossly, both human and porcine adult intestine are at a ratio of 0.1 length per kilogram of body weight. The anatomy of the small intestine is similar between pig and human, though the large intestine varies slightly in the pig due to a larger cecum, lack of appendix, and the presence of the spiral colon. Microscopically, for both species, the small and large intestine are comprised of a single layer of epithelial cells, interspersed with intra-epithelial lymphocytes, to serve as a barrier between luminal contents and systemic circulation. The single layer epithelium covers villus projections (present only in small intestine) and extends down into the crypts of Lieberkuhn. Located at the crypt-base are the intestinal epithelial stem cells (ISCs), which are responsible for renewing the epithelial cell populations on a continuous 3—5 day cycle). In the human, the ISCs are interspersed with Paneth cells, a specialized secretory cell type that both supports ISC function and releases antimicrobial factors into the intestinal lumen.

4. Beneath the epithelial barrier is the lamina propria compartment. While the lamina propria is made up of a mix of structural elements including blood and lymph vessels, connective tissue, and mesenchymal cells, immune cells constitute a major population, including dendritic cells and lymphocytes. These immune cells are responsible for discriminating between harmless luminal antigens and potential enteropathogens. Some differences exist between the immunologic organization between human and pig intestine such as the distribution and frequency of lamina propria and intraepithelial lymphocyte populations, the inverted structure of porcine peripheral and gut-associated lymph nodes, and the aggregated lymphoid follicles

which form one long continuous band in the porcine ileum. However, despite these differences, pigs are still recognized as useful models in several enteric immunologic studies including infectious disease, oral vaccination, small bowel transplantation, food hypersensitivity, and immune development.

5. With these similarities in both physiology and architecture between human and porcine intestine（猪小肠）, porcine models of various intestinal injuries such as ischemia-reperfusion injury（缺血再灌注损伤）, intestinal transplantation, short gut syndrome, and necrotizing enterocolitis have progressed the field of gastroenterology. Furthermore, in vitro advancements continue to broaden the utility of porcine enteric disease models. These advancements include an increase in porcine specific reagents and the use of primary intestinal epithelial cell culture in 2-D monolayers, 3-D organoid culture, and co-culture with microbes and laminapropria derived cells to better understand intestinal barrier function. However, for more mechanistic studies and to better understand human genetic diseases in the wide array of intestinal maladies, advancements in porcine gene-edited models are needed. Fortunately, enhanced strategies to edit the porcine genome and develop transgenic models, as well as approaches to genetically modify porcine-derived intestinal organoids, have increased the availability of pre-clinical modeling for Cystic Fibrosis (CF)（囊性纤维化）, colorectal cancer (CRC)（结肠直肠癌）, and ischemia-reperfusion injury. This review summarizes the current use of pre-clinical, gene edited porcine intestinal disease and injury models and evaluates future additional needs to ultimately improve treatment of intestinal disease.

6. Cystic Fibrosis (CF) is a life-threatening disease due to various mutations in the CF transmembrane conductance regulator（跨膜电导调节因子）(CFTR) gene. This critical gene encodes for an anion channel widely expressed in epithelium including lung, pancreas, kidney, and intestine; its loss of function inhibits chloride and bicarbonate transport across cell membranes. This leads to thick mucoid secretions with low pH, subsequent pathogen colonization, and dysregulated inflammation（失调性炎症）. While cause of death in patients afflicted with CF is primarily due to respiratory failure, intestinal disease also contributes significantly to patient morbidity. Up to 20% of infants with CF suffer from meconium ileus at birth, followed by distal intestinal obstructive syndrome due to intestinal atresia, diverticulosis, and microcolon. While genetically modified murine models of CF assisted in basic understanding of CFTR functions, these mice fail to fully recreate human clinical disease. These limitations in the mouse models impeded further discovery of disease pathogenesis and potential therapeutics.

7. In 2008, in an effort to develop an animal model that better represents CF clinical disease, Rogers et al. utilized recombinant adeno-associated virus (rAAV)（重组腺相关病毒）vectors to create the first CFTR-null piglets (CFTR-/-). These piglets

also demonstrated immediate clinical signs of intestinal obstruction similar to that in human infants with CF. These clinical signs include intestinal atresia, microcolon, and diverticulosis. Other gene editing strategies have since been used to generate CFTR-/- pigs including bacterial artificial chromosome vectors as well as rAAVs to introduce a point mutation within the CFTR gene, CFTR-OF508 mutation. This specific CFTR mutation is the most common CF-causing mutation in human patients—it accounts for about 70% of CF alleles. Murine models with this same induced point mutation fail to develop airway disease, pushing the need for a porcine model of this common mutation. While CFTR-OF508 porcine models display the same features of human disease in the lung and intestine, the rate of meconium ileus is 100% in the newborn pigs, in contrast to a rate of 20% in human infants. As in humans, meconium ileus requires immediate medical and/or surgical correction, which inhibited the use of the porcine model due to cost and complexity. These factors pushed researchers to utilize additional gene editing techniques to alleviate meconium ileus in the porcine model. Stoltz et al. were able to correct this phenotype by inducing CFTR expression under the control of intestinal fatty acid-binding protein (iFABP)（肠道脂肪酸结合蛋白）in CFTR-/- pig fibroblasts. These findings indicated that correcting the expression of CFTR by gene editing in the intestine is sufficient to prevent intestinal obstruction. Further work in the porcine CF models is necessary to identify exactly how much CFTR function is required for proper intestinal function.

8. Colorectal cancer（CRC）is the second leading cause of cancer related deaths for men and women combined. For many patients, including those with precursor familial adenomatous polyposis（FAP）（家族性腺瘤性息肉病）condition，CRC begins with germline or somatic mutations in the tumorsuppressor, adenomatous polyposis coli（APC）（结肠腺瘤性息肉病）gene. This key driver mutation initiates polyp formation in the colonic epithelium.

From Frontiers in Veterinary Science，2022（9）：878952

After reading

Task 8　Build your vocabulary.

Directions: Match the following words with their corresponding definitions and Chinese equivalents.

English: gastrointestinal therapeutics omnivorous longitudinal intestine continuous epithelia mechanistic expenditure immunology anatomy lamina

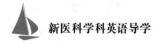

Chinese：胃小肠的　治疗法　杂食的　纵向的　肠　连续不断的　上皮细胞　机械论的
消耗　免疫学　解剖　薄层

Paras. 1—8

English	Chinese	Definition
1. _____	_____	a. of or related to the stomach and intestines
2. _____	_____	b. the branch of medicine concerned with the treatment of diseases
3. _____	_____	c. eating all types of food，especially both plants and meat
4. _____	_____	d. going downwards rather than across
5. _____	_____	e. a long tube in the body between the stomach and the anus. Food passes from the stomach to the small intestine and from there to the large intestine.
6. _____	_____	f. happening or existing for a period of time without interruption
7. _____	_____	g. membranous tissue covering internal organs and other internal surfaces of the body
8. _____	_____	h. connected with the belief that all things in the universe can be explained as if they were machines
9. _____	_____	i. the use of energy，time，materials，etc.
10. _____	_____	j. the scientific study of protection against disease
11. _____	_____	k. the structure of an animal or a plant
12. _____	_____	l. a thin plate or layer（especially of bone or mineral）

Guiding to learn

Task 9　Learn the following general academic vocabulary from the word bank.

conform features alternatively communication perspective principal coordinate
terminal minimal minority complexity sequence generate sequence transmission
theoretical modified coupled enforced dynamics dimensional emergent
framework

Beginning to read

Task 10　Now read the text.

Text C

Translational Neuronal Ensembles: Neuronal Microcircuits in Psychology, Physiology, Pharmacology and Pathology

Esther Lara-González et al

1. Nephrons, lobules, alveoli, acini and so forth work as functional units in body organs: multicellular organizations coordinating the actions of different cell classes to receive an input and yield and output, modules commonly ordered in tandem in a given organ and being preserved along the vertebrate phylogeny(脊椎动物系统发育). One advantage of these modular architecture is obvious: degradation of an organ due to degenerative chronic disorders or age, is a gradual steady decline before a complete failure is reached. The advent of multicellular recording techniques(多细胞记录技术的出现)has shown that many areas of the nervous system have a modular organization of neuronal populations, previously shown indirectly with intra-and extra-cellular unitary recordings associated with local field potentials and other population recordings: groups of neurons that coordinate themselves to work together in several brain areas to perform their functions have been defined as "canonical" microcircuits in Shepherd and Grillner (2018). A new advantage for experimentalists is that territorial coordinates of unitary activity while using multielectrode arrays (MEAs)(多电极阵列), or various neurons themselves using calcium imaging, can be identified, and followed within and without their groups with single cell resolution and be compared with population recordings. These findings ended a long debate about the functional unit of the nervous system: either the neuron or neuronal populations. In many brain areas, the functional units are neuronal ensembles: groups of coactive neurons.

2. There are many classes of neurons with their proper biophysical, biochemical and genetical features, however, in many areas of the brain, immunostaining(免疫染色), in situ hybridization(原位杂交), single cell PCR, transcriptomics and whole cell recordings have shown iterative modules accomplishing coordinated tasks. In a brief simplification, minimal features of a canonical microcircuit are: a group of GABAergic interneurons innervate principal neurons mainly in the dendrites and spines to control afferent inputs and feed-back entries, while other groups of interneurons mainly innervate the perisomatic area and axon hillock to control

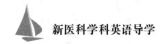

principal neurons output. Principal cells are surrounded by these interneurons controlling input and output in a consensual trait，plus interconnections between principal neurons and long-range interneurons form feed-forward networks including disinhibition. Perhaps recording of thousands of neurons (Stringer et al.，2021) show only the tip of the iceberg. Alternatively，scalability shows similar sequence patterns from the histological scale（dozens of neurons）to the mesoscale（hundreds of neurons）. Regular modular elements with similar electrophysiological profiles and markers expression can be found in all cortical mantles including the hippocampus，the striatal circuit（纹状体回路），and with slightly different profiles and names the cerebellum. Importantly，they resonate at different frequencies and are main components of cerebral oscillations（脑振荡）and rhythms generation，which could be a way of additional communication besides axons，terminals and volume transmission.

3. An important factor to understand the association of particular neuron types and their cuasi-iterative prevalence（准迭代发病率） is of course programmed embryogenesis（Li et al.，2016）. In addition，there is the theoretical framework synthesized by Hebb（1949）and later modified with experiments from numerous groups. Although the generic name for these modules may be："neuronal ensembles"（神经元集合），their composition and complete numbers in different contexts is unknown. For example，by identifying and following samples of motor cortical ensembles in vitro at histological level it was found that most sampled ensembles have PV + neurons (Serrano-Reyes et al.，2020). Similar experiments must be done with the different kinds of interneurons and principal cells（Markram et al.，2015）to describe their composition and observe their dynamics，since ensembles are composed with inhibitory and principal neurons playing various roles. Due to these cited experiments，to simplify the cellular-synaptic complexity（细胞突触的复杂性）and make sense at the network level，neuronal ensembles，defined as "groups of neurons that show spatiotemporal co-activation"（显示时空共激活的神经元群）（Yuste，2015） are commonly linked with "functional connectivities" between recording sites while using multi-recording techniques. Dimensional reduction（降维）can be used to position ensembles in a neuronal state space（Ebitz and Hayden，2021）. Neurons with correlated firing are sorted together by functional connections and their activity alternates due to connections between ensembles，which can be illustrated as trajectories in low-dimensional space and connectivity graphs（Calderón et al.，2022）. This simplification allows going from the cellular-synaptic level to the emergent properties of recorded networks（Carrillo-Reid et al.，2015）：in a "bottom-up" direction.

From Frontiers in Systems Neuroscience，*2022（1）：979680*

New words and expressions

coordinate /kəʊˈɔːdɪneɪt，kəʊˈɔːdɪnət/ *vt*. to organize the different parts of an activity and the people involved in it so that it works well 使协调;使相配合

microcircuit /ˈmaɪkrəʊˌsɜːkət/ *n*. a microelectronic computer circuit incorporated into a chip or semiconductor 微型电路

computational /ˌkɒmpjʊˈteɪʃənl/ *adj*. using or connected with computers 使用计算机的; 与计算机有关的

hypothesis /haɪˈpɒθəsɪs/ *n*. an idea or explanation of sth that is based on a few known facts but that has not yet been proved to be true or correct(有少量事实依据但未被证实的)假说;假设

degradation /ˌdegrəˈdeɪʃn/ *n*. process of something becoming worse or weaker 恶化

territorial /ˌterəˈtɔːriəl/ *adj*. connected with the land or sea that is owned by a particular country 领土的;地盘性的

connectivity /ˌkɒnekˈtɪvəti/ *n*. the state of being connected or the degree to which two things are connected 连接(度);联结(度)

speculative /ˈspekjələtɪv/ *adj*. based on guessing or on opinions that have been formed without knowing all the facts 推测的;猜测的;推断的

canonical /kəˈnɒnɪkl/ *adj*. connected with works of literature that are highly respected 经典的;标准的

hybridization /ˌhaɪbrɪdaɪˈzeɪʃn/ *n*. (genetics) the act of mixing different species or varieties of animals or plants and thus to produce hybrids 杂化;杂混;杂交

resonate /ˈrezəneɪt/ *v*. (of a voice，an instrument，etc.) to make a deep, clear sound that continues for a long time 产生共鸣;发出回响

After reading

Task 11　Build your vocabulary. Choose one word which can be used to replace the language shown in bold without changing the meaning of the sentence from the list below. Change forms and cases when necessary.

activist(*n*.)　assist(*v*.)　clarify(*v*.)　converse(*v*.)　extract(*v*.)　incline(*v*.) propagate(*v*.)　propensity(*n*.)　sustain(*v*.)　urban(*adj*.)

1. A closer examination of the central and peripheral effects of leptin will **explain** its observed role in CVD progression more clearly. ＿＿＿＿＿＿＿＿

2. Swiftly，the pedagogical focus has translated into a social agenda in the research field，motivating both theoretical and empirical efforts that inspire and **grow** one another. ＿＿＿＿＿＿＿＿

3. But the **talk** can also be true; it is possible that the unknown threshold is not reached, in which case the putative transfer will not occur, leaving a child weak in both languages, and thus become even more disadvantaged.

4. Instead, participants were more **disposed** counter a personal threat by enhancing their ingroup, a strategy quite in keeping with the tenets of social identity theory.

5. Policy changes, economic support and improved participatory design techniques can **help** with effective community revitalization.

6. That corruption **takes out** half of education budget means that the DepEd Can theoretically have twice the resources available to schools, teachers, and students.

7. Thus this human feedback from infected individuals to aquatic reservoirs appears critical to **maintain** the so-called primary transmission, which underscores the importance of secondary transmission itself.

8. It is also caused by once rural populations' migration to **inner-city** regions, where a dense human population is prime for vector transmission of the disease.

9. A chemotaxis assay that examined the **tendency** of VSMC to migrate towards a chemoattractant solution of leptin through a microchemotaxis chamber revealed that 3 fold more cells were able to migrate through a polycarbonate membrane following a leptin trail than with no leptin trail.

10. On principle, this sounds rather elementary, but looking at a field like conservation or even an issue like education, policymakers and **campaigners** are both campaigning very strongly to maintain or improve their sector, even if nothing is yet going wrong.

Further reading

Augustin, R. C., Leone, R. D., Naing A, et al. (2022). Next Steps for Clinical Translation of Adenosine Pathway Inhibition in Cancer Immunotherapy. *Journal for Immunotherapy of Cancer*. 10(2).

Lara-González, E., Padilla-Orozco, M., Fuentes-Serrano, A., et al.(2022). Translational Neuronal Ensembles: Neuronal Microcircuits in Psychology, Physiology, Pharmacology and Pathology. *Frontiers in Systems Neuroscience*. Aug 24.

Sims, S. K., Wilken-Resman, B., Smith, C. J., et al. (2022). Brain-Derived Neurotrophic Factor and Nerve Growth Factor Therapeutics for Brain Injury: The Current Translational Challenges in Preclinical and Clinical Research. *Neural Plasticity*. Mar 2.

Zhou, Y., Xu, J., Hou, Y., et al. (2022). The Alzheimer's Cell Atlas (TACA): A Single-Cell Molecular Map for Translational Therapeutics Accelerator in Alzheimer's Disease. *Alzheimer's & Dementia: Translational Research & Clinical Interventions* (N Y). 8(1).

Unit 7
Clinical Practice and Translational Medicine

Guiding to learn

When it comes to health and disease, we can not escape it. Disease is due to the existence of disease genes or external environmental stimuli in the genetic system in the body, which act on the cells in the body, cause or induce harmful changes in life function, and make the body metabolism and function occur abnormal. Although the most intuitive damage to the disease is for the body, but the psychological damage can not be ignored. Therefore, learning about these severe diseases is significant for people.

Discuss the following questions with your partners.

1. What is the aim of translational and implementation sciences?
2. What is the Marfan syndrome?
3. What is the Alzheimer's disease?

Task 1   Learn the following general academic vocabulary.

available conception   identification   indicate   responsive   community
traditionally   commentary   corresponding   exclusively   proportion
implementation   integration   investigator   professional promote consultant
facilitator   sustainability   enhance   expertise   innovation   intervention
appreciable   preliminary   conceive persistent

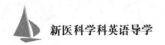

Beginning to read

Task 2　Now read the text.

Text A

Advancing Translation of Clinical Research Into Practice and Population Health Impact Through Implementation Science
Lila J. Finney Rutten et al

1. RESEARCH TO PRACTICE GAP

The gap between establishing scientific evidence and integrating that evidence into routine clinical practice has been well characterized. It is frequently noted that only a small proportion of scientific innovation is translated into routine clinical practice and that even then, the process can take more than a decade. Whereas this lag may vary by measurement approach, funding mechanism, and other factors, more recently published estimates indicate that it takes an average of 14 years and $2 billion to bring a new drug or medical device from conception to market. This research-to-practice gap has not historically been an important consideration in academic clinical research. The clinical research enterprise typically rewards the conduct of descriptive or mechanistic studies that are highly controlled. Although growing attention has focused on the need to accelerate translation of knowledge into clinical practice, protocolized intervention trials（协议化干预试验）for evidence generation are often designed without appreciable attention paid to evidence translation and therefore do not lend themselves to integration of innovation into feasible and sustainable health care programs and policies in real world settings. Integration of translational and implementation science（转化和实施科学）principles and practices into clinical research can advance the translation of scientific innovation into improved patient care and population health.

2. DEFINING TRANSLATION, TRANSLATIONAL RESEARCH, AND TRANSLATIONAL SCIENCE

Adopting relevant terminology and definitions of the National Center for Advancing Translational Sciences throughout this commentary, we refer to the broad goal of moving scientific innovation into routine clinical practice and population health impact as translation; to the specific process of conducting research in a manner to support movement between the phases of the translational continuum（转化连续体）, translational research; and last, to the disciplinary field of study and resultant body of general operative evidence，translational science.

3. TRANSLATIONAL SCIENCE CONTINUUM

Translational research occurs along a continuum of scientific innovation that includes 5 phases of research（T0 to T4），from basic biologic or behavioral research （T0 to T2）to research with humans，patients，clinical practices，and communities（T3 and T4）. The translational science continuum（转化科学连续体）highlights the specific outcomes of research in each phase，with a corresponding continuum of clinical trial designs from explanatory to pragmatic，depending on the type of evidence generation required. Increasingly，translational science is being extended beyond the bedside to have an impact on routine clinical practice and population health. The translational science continuum thus represents a broad "bench-to-bedside"（从实验室到临床） movement of discoveries from the controlled research laboratory to routine clinical or community settings（社区环境）. Investments in the clinical and translational sciences， including those by the National Institutes of Health，are intended to accelerate translational research through each phase of translation. Translational roadblocks（转 化障碍）have been characterized as occurring between specific phases of the translational continuum，emphasizing the challenges or translational blocks occurring between animal and first-in-human studies（首次在人体试验），efficacy and effectiveness trials，and identification of evidence-based practice and its use in routine care. These roadblocks，which arise in part because of the professional and scientific silos that distinguish each research phase，serve to deter or slow progression from basic scientific discoveries to population health impact. Using transdisciplinary research and team science，translational science seeks to identify and address these roadblocks in translation and to create efficiencies to accelerate the integration of biomedical innovation into applications that improve population health. To this end，the scientific principles of translational science include a focus on addressing unmet patient，clinic， community，or population needs and emphasize creating generalizable solutions to persistent challenges in translation of innovation into practice. Major funding organizations have in recent years created funding opportunities to incentivize translational team science focused on addressing unmet needs and creating and evaluating sustainable and scalable solutions to improve patient care and population health. For example，the authors of this review are members of teams leading 2 such efforts. The first is a pragmatic trial（实用的实验）with process evaluation of patient- and provider-facing interventions to increase human papillomavirus vaccination rates （乳头瘤病毒接种率）.The objective is to move evidence based vaccines，reported to be efficacious in randomized clinical trials（随机临床试验），into routine clinical practice and family settings. The second is a pragmatic trial with process evaluation of a guideline-informed enhanced，electronic health record-facilitated cancer symptom control care model that aims to integrate evidence-based approaches to cancer symptom management into clinical workflows and to make them available to patients between clinical encounters. These efforts, led by transdisciplinary teams inclusive of clinical, epidemiologic, implementation science, and behavioral science experts, aim to understand and to improve the delivery of evidence-based care（循证医学）and to improve population health and are examples of research focused on translation to practice（T3）and translation to community（T4）.

4. DEFINING IMPLEMENTATION, IMPLEMENTATION RESEARCH, AND IMPLEMENTATION SCIENCE

A powerful approach to characterize and to address translational roadblocks is through application of the principles and practices of implementation science. Implementation science is the scientific discipline focused on "methods to promote the systematic uptake of research findings and other evidence-based practices into routine practice, and, hence, to improve the quality and effectiveness of health services". The National Institutes of Health defines implementation as "the process of putting to use or integrating evidence-based interventions（基于证据的干预措施）within a setting" and describes implementation research as study of "the processes and factors that are associated with successful integration of evidence-based interventions within a particular setting". Implementation science frequently seeks to test and to apply practices and approaches that increase adoption and sustainment of evidence-based interventions into routine clinical care（常规临床护理）. By identifying multilevel barriers to and facilitators of evidence based practices in routine clinical care, implementation science develops, applies, and evaluates targeted strategies across multiple levels（patient, provider, care team, system）to increase adoption and to support sustainability of evidence-based practices. Whereas implementation is often conceived of as occurring during final stages of the translational science continuum, the principles and practices of implementation science can be usefully applied across the translational continuum to support movement across the translational phases. Indeed, implementation science has been described as a "sub-science"（科学分支）of translational science wherein the principles and practices of implementation science can be applied to identify, investigate, and systematically apply strategies to proactively accelerate translation of scientific innovation into routine clinical practice and population impact. Use of a "design with implementation in mind" approach for clinical trials across translational stages can address translational roadblocks earlier in the research continuum and advance the translation of innovation into practice, especially the roadblocks encountered between late-stage trials（后期实验）and adoption in routine clinical practice or population settings.

5. APPLYING IMPLEMENTATION SCIENCE IN CLINICAL TRIALS TO ADVANCE TRANSLATION

Funding agencies are increasingly encouraging transdisciplinary team science drawing on the principles and practices of implementation science to ensure greater return on funding investments in clinical research. To be responsive to funding opportunities and to increase the impact of their research efforts, clinical research teams who have traditionally focused exclusively or primarily on T1 and T2 trials are increasingly seeking out implementation scientists and integrating implementation science into study designs. Various approaches for including implementation scientists in research have been summarized, and the approach often depends on the aims of the relevant research. For example, an implementation scientist may serve as a consultant, an advisory board member, or coinvestigator to inform exploratory or preliminary aims focused on context evaluation, to assess implementation outcomes, or to inform implementation or dissemination strategy. Implementation scientists may also lead aims that are specifically focused on development, tailoring, and evaluation of implementation strategies. They may also serve as principal investigator of efforts wherein the primary aim is specific to dissemination and implementation science or co-lead research efforts in a multipl-principal investigator arrangement bringing together clinical or public health expertise with implementation science expertise to improve delivery of evidence-based practice(循证实践) in clinical and community settings.

From Mayo Clinic Proceedings，2024，99(4)

New words and expressions

resultant /rɪˈzʌltənt/ *adj*. caused by the thing that has just been mentioned 因而发生的；因此而产生的

roadblock /ˈrəʊdblɒk/ *n*. any condition that makes it difficult to make progress or to achieve an objective 障碍

transdisciplinary /træns'dɪsəplɪnəri/ *adj*. cross－disciplinary 跨学科的；学科间的

incentivize /ɪnˈsentɪvaɪz/ *v*. to provide (someone) with a good reason for wanting to do something 激励(某人做某事)

unmet /ˌʌnˈmet/ *adj*. not satisfied 未满足的

scalable /ˈskeɪləbl/ *adj*. capable of being expanded or climbed 可扩展的

vaccination /ˌvæksɪˈneɪʃ(ə)n/ *n*. taking a vaccine as a precaution against contracting a disease 接种疫苗，种痘

epidemiologic /ˈepɪˌdiːmɪəˈlɒdʒɪk/ *adj*. of or relating to epidemiology 流行病学的；传染病学的

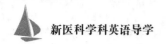

After reading

Task 3　Read Text A again and answer the following questions.

1. How much do you know about the translational science continuum?

2. What is your understanding of implementation science? How to apply implementation science in clinical trials to advance translation?

Task 4　Check your vocabulary. Fill in the blanks with the correct form of the words from the following box, each word can be used only once.

adolescent (*n.*)　affiliate (*v.*)　aristocracy (*n.*)　cell (*n.*)　collapse (*n.*) commodity(*n.*)　democracy(*n.*)　dissolve(*v.*)　friction(*n.*)　invoke(*v.*)　muscle(*n.*) repudiate(*v.*)　saint(*n.*)

1. Conversely, fetal leptin may actually make fetal insulin more sensitive to glucose usage, stimulating _____ growth.

2. There are five Healthy People 2010 objectives that relate to _____ diabetes.

3. In addition to deaths, Malaria causes a multitude of complications and disease to those who do not die from infection: seizures, coma, severe anemia, pulmonary edema, thrombocytopenia, cardiovascular _____ , shock, acute kidney failure, and hypoglycemia.

4. Friction is an important factor of workers' ability to grasp and manipulate work objects and their risks of developing work related musculoskeletal disorders (MSDs), since poor _____ conditions require greater grip force to prevent slipping of objects, and repetitive forceful exertions, common in industries, are well known as the cause of MSDs.

5. The bill will benefit our nations economy because ethanol can help stabilize _____ prices, provide competition, increase net farm income, boosts employment and improve the equilibrium of trade.

6. Considering that Benjamin is a longstanding _____ and once high-level leader of the AAUP, it should come to no surprise that he has motives to preserve the distinction, honor, and prestige of the faculty profession.

7. DNA was extracted from fin clips, or from _____ tissue from the right side of the specimen using Proteinase K dissolution.

8. Through upwelling and downwelling, these gasses are transitioned to and from the surface layer, from whence they _____ into and out of the atmosphere.

9. This will _____ the feel-nothing reading. Once that is out of the way, we can finish up with my own proposal.

10. Furthermore, each explicit prime is designed to _____ a threat that both paired groups share.

Task 5   Build your vocabulary. Read the sentences below, decide which word in each bracket is more suitable.

1. The effects of ingestion include nausea, vomiting, diarrhea, convulsions, (depressed/distressed) respiration and more, including death in some cases.

2. However, the streetcar lines that Droege referred to were (antique/obsolete) by 1956, overtaken by bus and automobile transport.

3. The process eliminates (odour/fragrance) and accelerates decomposition.

4. It took a long time to (refute/contradict) these claims with evidence of the safety and benefits of midwifery.

5. There is a place on the worksheet to fill out the taste, (texture/touch), color, and whether or not the child likes that particular food.

6. As can be seen, removal projects are not always (dogmatic/pragmatic) or even possible.

7. However, despite the influence of structural violence the (incessant/eternal) rise of HIV and MTCT rates is also due to the failure of intercepting initiatives to tackle transmission.

8. A strong connection was observed between location of the streams and habitat assessment (scores/results).

9. Mexico and the Philippines have both concluded agreements with their commercial bank (debtors/creditors).

10. Cross A F1 females all inherit one copy of the wild type eye color gene which is enough to (discuss/confer) the wild type phenotype so eye color is a recessive trait.

Guiding to learn

Task 6   Learn the following general academic vocabulary.

assessment evident identification specificity maintain previously transfer
considerable criterion outcome reliability sequence contrast summary
fundamental stability neutralization underlying classical detection intensive
spontaneous matate obstacle

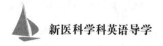

Beginning to read

Task 7　Now read the text.

Text B

Translational Medicine in Hereditary Hemorrhagic Telangiectasia
Riera-Mestre A et al

1. Hereditary hemorrhagic telangiectasia（HHT）（遗传性出血性毛细血管扩张症）or Rendu-Osler-Weber syndrome is a rare autosomal dominant vascular disease characterized by systemic telangiectases（毛细血管扩张）and larger vascular malformations（VMs）（血管畸形）. The hallmark of HHT is telangiectasis，which are dilated postcapillary venules directly connected with dilated arterioles losing the capillary bed. HHT can be diagnosed either using the Curaçao clinical criteria or through molecular genetic test. Mutations in the endoglin（ENG）and activin（激活素）A receptor type II-like 1（ACVRL1）genes are detected in approximately 90% of cases submitted for molecular diagnosis and cause HHT1 and HHT2，respectively. Endoglin（encoded by ENG）is an auxiliary co-receptor at the endothelial cell（EC）surface that promotes BMP9（Bone morphogenetic protein 9）signaling through the activin receptor-like kinase 1（ALK1；encoded by ACVRL1）. Thus，HHT is now considered a disease of the hub formed by BMP9 – Endoglin – ALK1 – Smad，rather than a disease of the TGFB pathway.

2. Although many HHT features have been elucidated，there are still several questions that remain unsolved. It is unknown why telangiectases are typically found in characteristics sites，as in fingertips of the hands or nasal mucosa（causing recurrent epistaxis，which are the most frequent clinical manifestation）or the reason why pulmonary arteriovenous malformations（AVMs）（动静脉畸形）are more common in patients with HHT1 and hepatic VMs in HHT2. Also，the genetic landscape of HHT is unclear，as there are 10%—15% of patients with HHT phenotype who are genetically orphan. Moreover，despite showing equal pathogenic variants，there is high inter-and intra-familial variability in vascular involvement and clinical manifestations. Another unsolved question is that，in spite HHT is a congenital condition，it exhibits an age-related penetrance as epistaxis is the earliest clinical manifestation and most patients have developed larger VMs before 40 years but surprisingly，gastrointestinal bleeding symptoms usually develop at fifth or sixth decades. Moreover，the low prevalence and

high clinical variability make understanding HHT a challenge，especially in uncommon situations. Together，these unresolved questions have hampered the development of a curative therapy for HHT patients. Thus，increasing understanding of HHT is vital for providing insights into molecular regulation of vascular development and improving care of patients.

3. The European Society for Translational Medicine （EUSTM） defined Translational Medicine（TM）in 2015 as "an interdisciplinary branch of the biomedical field supported by three main pillars：benchside，bedside，and community. The goal of TM is to combine disciplines，resources，expertise，and techniques within these pillars to promote enhancements in prevention，diagnosis，and therapies". Accordingly，a multidisciplinary approach is essential in TM and correlates indeed，with the importance of a multidisciplinary medical team when dealing with patients affected by rare diseases，such as HHT. TM must depart from medical attention to patients，so this multidisciplinary team should be the starting point. Because of clinical research difficulties in rare diseases，including basic research is crucial to improve management of these patients. However，there is usually a wide gap in the transition between preclinical （"basic"） and clinical stages because basic experiments may not reflect the real patients' demands. Thus，TM seems a good strategy to bring the two types of research closer as it implies both，clinical and basic researchers，working together. In fact，the adjective "translational" refers to the transference of the basic scientific findings from a laboratory setting into a clinical one. This is not only important as a way to get new discoveries，but also to enhance bench-to-bedside transition. The aim of this review is to exhibit some of the benefits that TM provide to HHT patients management，as a disease's model.

From European Journal of Internal Medicine，*2022*，*95*，*32 - 37*

After reading

Task 8   Build your vocabulary.

Directions：Match the following words with their corresponding definitions and Chinese equivalents.

English：elucidate   complication   diagnosis   congenital   armamentarium
Chinese：先天的   解释   诊断   医疗设备   并发症

Paras. 1—2

English	Chinese	Definition
1. _____	_____	a. existing since or before birth
2. _____	_____	b. make clear and（more）comprehensible
3. _____	_____	c. identifying the nature or cause of some phenomenon
4. _____	_____	d. the collection of equipment and methods used in the practice of medicine
5. _____	_____	e. any disease or disorder that occurs during the course of (or because of) another disease

English：density preclinical specificity permanent transference
Chinese：永久的 潜伏期的 ［免疫］特异性 转移 密度

Paras. 2—3

English	Chinese	Definition
6. _____	_____	f. continuing or enduring without marked change in status or condition or place
7. _____	_____	g. of or relating to the early phases of a disease when accurate diagnosis is not possible because symptoms of the disease have not yet appeared
8. _____	_____	h. the quality of being specific to a particular organism
9. _____	_____	i. the process of moving sth from one place, person or use to another
10. _____	_____	j. the amount per unit size

Guiding to learn

Task 9 Learn the following general academic vocabulary from the word bank.

> domain research aggregated fundamental individual validated accumulation
> highlight constantly assessed identify sufficiently investigation detected
> participant incorporated differentiate widespread structural emerge processing
> concluding accurate technology furthermore priority interventions implication
> maintain differentiate specific stability functional crucially

Beginning to read

Task 10　Now read the text.

Text C

Science Disconnected: The Translational Gap between Basic Science, Clinical trials, and Patient care in Alzheimer's Disease

Sarah Gregory et al

1. Alois Alzheimer discovered the soon-to-become eponymous condition of Alzheimer's disease（阿尔茨海默病）in 1906, describing misfolded and then aggregated amyloid β and tau, brain atrophy, and a host of cognitive and functional symptoms. Accordingly, clinical symptoms of memory loss formed a prominent, and then core, part of the diagnostic criteria for Alzheimer's disease, alongside functional impairment. With clinical history and neuropsychological（神经心理学）assessment forming the basis of Alzheimer's disease investigations throughout the 20th century, Alzheimer's disease became predominantly conceptualised as a cognitive disorder due to its late-stage clinical manifestations. Despite advancements in in-vivo biomarker development to support diagnosis, this legacy of considering Alzheimer's disease mainly in the context of cognition is proving resilient, hampering clinical practice（妨碍临床实践）and clinical trials. As such, the majority of clinical trial work has been done with people in the very late, symptomatic or dementia phases（老年痴呆阶段）of the disease. We now know that there is a long, silent (or preclinical) period of Alzheimer's disease, beginning as early as midlife (40—65 years of age), followed by a shorter prodromal period (3—6 years before symptom onset). Both the preclinical and prodromal periods could represent key windows for interventions to delay or even prevent dementia. Crucially, the period currently conceptualised as being silent (or asymptomatic) is becoming increasingly detectable through biomarker discovery and development. Importantly, during these periods, cognitive symptoms are largely absent. Thereby, it might be time to revisit Alois Alzheimer's original proposal of Alzheimer's as a brain disease, which might be more readily detected in its early stages using new biomarkers, rather than continue its classification as a syndromal cognitive disorder（综合征性认知障碍）.

2. There are three overarching considerations for the planning of future trials in Alzheimer's disease: (1) the right disease pathology target; (2) the right time in the

disease process; and (3) the right person. The trial population needs to be sufficiently phenotyped to identify individuals at each disease stage. We will discuss recent developments in the field of Alzheimer's disease that inform each of these stages and argue for a triad approach to Alzheimer's disease clinical trials that would further enhance all three. In terms of selecting the right participants, we will also highlight developments in the brain health clinic service (脑部健康诊所服务), which is a necessary upstream requirement to support more targeted clinical trial efforts.

3. The field of biomarker discovery for Alzheimer's disease is constantly evolving. Many clinical trials of prodromal Alzheimer's disease now include metabolic measures, such as PET imaging, either as screening tools for study eligibility or as secondary or tertiary outcome measures. Currently, a PET tracer compound is being developed to detect synaptic loss, which is a crucial event in Alzheimer's disease pathology thought to correspond with the start of observable cognitive impairment and other behavioural and neuropsychiatric problems. The early onset of cognitive impairment is also when most patients first present to clinical services and thereafter enter into research studies, albeit in smaller numbers. Although this radiotracer has not yet been verified in autopsy studies, synaptic loss has been well correlated with cognitive decline in previous post-mortem investigations, suggesting that this measure is likely to be a useful biomarker in the future. Regarding neuroimaging, recent focus has been on the thinning of certain brain regions, such as hippocampal subfields and the entorhinal cortex, as a highly sensitive measure of structural changes in the pre-dementia stages of Alzheimer's disease. Although promising, robust measurement techniques must be developed before these neuroimaging metrics can be incorporated into clinical trials as primary or secondary outcomes. Historically, the validation of biomarkers for Alzheimer's disease (eg, PET ligands and cerebrospinal fluid [CSF] assays) has been through autopsy studies. The incorporation of these in-vivo PET and CSF biomarkers into the diagnostic criteria for Alzheimer's disease in the National Institute on Aging-Alzheimer's Association Research Framework 2018 has led the Alzheimer's Precision Medicine Initiative Working Group to call for the validation of blood-based biomarkers for cognitive impairment. Evidence suggests that blood tests measuring amyloid $\beta 42$ to amyloid $\beta 40$ ratios correlate with cortical amyloid β deposition, with a positive predictive value of 81%. Similarly, plasma amyloid (血浆淀粉样蛋白) β measurements have been shown to have a high stability and sensitivity, suggesting that this metric could be used to detect Alzheimer's disease in its early stages now and as a screening test in the future. Additionally, measuring phosphorylated tau in the blood can predict tau and amyloid β pathologies, differentiate Alzheimer's disease from other neurodegenerative disorders, and identify Alzheimer's disease across the clinical continuum. As such, blood phosphorylated (血液磷酸化) tau shows particular potential as a less invasive, cost-effective biomarker of Alzheimer's disease pathology. Alongside

the more familiar amyloid and tau proteins，neurofilament(神经丝)light polypeptide is increasingly being considered a possible biomarker for Alzheimer's disease pathology. Once these novel neuroimaging(新型神经影像学) and biological biomarkers are validated，there will be no need to access specialists and specialist facilities for pre-screening in clinical trials，which could increase global access to studies. These metrics could also act as sensitive outcome measures.

From Lancet Healthy Longevity，2022，3(11)

New words and expressions

dementia /dɪˈmenʃə/ *n*. mental deterioration of organic or functional origin 痴呆，失智

prodromal /ˈprɒdrəʊməl/ *adj*. symptomatic of the onset of an attack or a disease 前驱的，有前驱症状的

polypeptide /ˌpɒlɪˈpeptaɪd/ *n*. a peptide containing 10 to more than 100 amino acids 多肽；缩多氨酸

neuronal /njʊəˈrəʊnəl/ *n*. of or relating to neurons 神经元的

disorder /dɪsˈɔːdə(r)/ *n*. a physical condition in which there is a disturbance of normal functioning 失调

neuropsychology /ˌnjʊərəʊsaɪˈkɒlədʒi/ *n*. the branch of psychology that is concerned with the physiological bases of psychological processes 神经心理学

inhibitor /ɪnˈhɪbɪtə(r)/ *n*. a substance that retards or stops an activity 抑制剂，抑制者；抗老化剂

monoclonal /ˌmɒnəʊˈkləʊnəl/ *adj*. forming or derived from a single clone 单克隆的

scopolamine /skəʊˈpɒləmiːn/ *n*. an alkaloid with anticholinergic effects that is used as a sedative and to treat nausea and to dilate the pupils in ophthalmic procedures 东莨菪碱(可用做镇静剂)

After reading

Task 11   **Build your vocabulary. Choose one word which can be used to replace the language shown in bold without changing the meaning of the sentence from the list below. Change forms and cases when necessary.**

alcohol(*n*.)	competence(*n*.)	conserve(*v*.)	corporate(*adj*.)	defer(*v*.)
domestic(*adj*.)	fraction(*n*.)	horror(*n*.)	incentive(*n*.)	negotiate(*v*.)
peasant(*n*.)	prudence(*n*.)	rhythm(*n*.)		

1. For the cardiovascular assessment，I heard his distinct irregularly irregular **beat** characteristic that of atrial fibrillation or atrial flutter with varying blocks.

2. This changed cows from **home** animals into meat-producing machines，raw material to be fed into the hungry capitalist monster that Chicago became as its meatpackers revolutionized consumption patterns in America. _____

3. However，the economic forest could not **protect** water and soil as effectively as the ecological forest do. _____

4. Regardless，as a future primary care provider，I should not **postpone** this or refer to an urologist until I have performed the examination. _____

5. Alternatively，they may see **inducements** for issuing fewer violations in order to meet this goal. _____

6. This example embodies the flaws inherent to **organizational** self regulation of health standards. _____

7. Yet even these numbers don't represent a **small proportion** of the global demand for forest products. _____

8. They do not consider the possibility that it might simply be the reaction of a curious and perhaps **dread** stricken child! _____

9. Jane should be cautioned to avoid **strong drink**，smoke，undercooked meat，raw eggs，sweeteners，and should be limited 1 - 2 cups caffeine. _____

10. However，since the casual relationship is often unclear，the authors argue **wisdom** when exploring speciation events based on these traits. _____

Further reading

Fonseca，A.，Lobo，J.，Hazard，F. K.，et al.（2022）. Advancing Clinical and Translational Research in Germ Cell Tumours（GCT）：Recommendations from the Malignant Germ Cell International Consortium. *British Journal of Cancer*. 127(9).

Gregory，S.，Saunders，S.，Ritchie，C. W.（2022）. Science Disconnected：The Translational Gap Between Basic Science，Clinical Trials，and Patient Care in Alzheimer's Disease. *Lancet Healthy Longevity*. 3(11).

Kallenbach，K.，Remes，A.，Müller，O. J.，et al.（2022）. Translational Medicine：Towards Gene Therapy of Marfan Syndrome. *Journal of Clinical Medicine*. 11(14).

Lauer，E. M.，Mutter，J.，Scherer，F.（2022）. Circulating Tumor DNA in B-cell lymphoma：Technical Advances，Clinical Applications，and Perspectives for Translational Research. *Leukemia*. 36(9).

Rutten，L. J. F.，Ridgeway，J. L.，& Griffin，J. M.（2024）. Advancing Translation of Clinical Research into Practice and Population Health Impact through Implementation Science. *Mayo Clinic Proceedings*. 99(4).

Unit 8
Artificial Intelligence in Translational Medicine

Guiding to learn

The opportunities and limitations around implementing AI-based methods in biomarker discovery and patient selection and how advances in digital pathology and AI should be considered in the current landscape of translational medicine are discussed. Artificial Intelligence and proteomics in transformational medicine of hepatocellular carcinoma is also discussed. Rapid accumulation of large-scale cancer omics data is catalysed by breakthroughs in high-throughput technologies. The current situation and future challenges of these data for promoting cancer research and treatment have also been studied.

Discuss the following questions with your partners.

1. What are the improvements gained from digital pathology?
2. What are basic data types in cancer research?
3. What is hepatocellular carcinoma?

Task 1 Learn the following general academic vocabulary.

assessment available consistent distribute inconsistency interpretation variability
acquisition administration appropriate computational distinct evaluation feature
perception regulatory relevant criteria document initially interaction maximize
accessible integration consultation entity facilitate generate margin orientation
transition accuracy initiation transport utility convert differentiate extract
unique automated crucial detection highlight unbiased

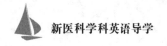

Beginning to read

Task 2   Now read the text.

Text A

Digital Pathology and Artificial Intelligence in Translational Medicine and Clinical Practice
Vipul Baxi et al

1. Pathology（病理学）has historically played a crucial role in the drug development process，including preclinical research to facilitate target identification，define drug mechanism of action and pharmacodynamics（药效学），and enable toxicology（毒理学）assessments. More recently，pathology has formed a bridge between drug discovery，translational，and clinical research programs that are striving to decipher disease pathophysiology（病理生理学）in the context of the mechanism of action，patient selection，or patient stratification. Such insights form the basis of novel hypotheses that can further be explored in drug discovery programs or applied to inform clinical trial design，thereby improving the probability of technical and regulatory success.

2. Pathology-based assessments have been used to classify disease and determine efficacy in drug development across a variety of disease areas. For example，during phase 2 trials for drug development in non-alcoholic steatohepatitis，the US Food and Drug Administration（FDA）（美国食品药品监督管理局）considers evidence of efficacy on a histological endpoint to support initiation of phase 3 trials. Additionally，pathological complete response（pCR）（病理完全缓解）has been studied as a surrogate endpoint in patients with cancer for the prediction of long-term clinical benefit and favorable prognosis with the administration of neoadjuvant therapy. More recently，pCR was associated with improved long-term efficacy in patients with human epidermal growth factor receptor 2 （HER2）-positive breast cancer treated with chemotherapy plus either intravenous or subcutaneous trastuzumab. In the immuno-oncology （I-O）（免疫肿瘤学）arena，immune-related pathologic response criteria have been applied retrospectively to surgical specimens from patients treated with immunotherapy in the neoadjuvant or advanced disease setting to predict survival in several tumor types.

3. Immunohistochemistry（IHC）（免疫组织化学）has been used to characterize

biomarkers, such as programmed cell death-ligand 1 (PD-L1)(程序性细胞死亡配体 1), and their association with clinical benefit. Traditional pathology techniques present several advantages, such as low cost, widespread availability, and application on formalin-fixed, paraffinembedded (FFPE) tissue samples, but challenges pertaining to differences in laboratory methods and subjective interpretation, particularly with the evaluation of immune cell staining, may lead to inter-observer variability. This can produce inconsistency in diagnoses, which may impact treatment decisions. While the use of IHC assays has led to better identification of patients who respond to I-O therapy, there remains a need to more accurately quantify complex immune markers, including cell phenotypes in a spatial context, that require advanced quantitative tools to maximize the amount of information yielded from individual samples.

4. Artificial intelligence (AI) applications in pathology improve quantitative accuracy and enable the geographical contextualization of data using spatial algorithms. Adding spatial metrics to IHC can improve the clinical value of biomarker identification approaches. For example, in a recent meta-analysis, the addition of spatial context to IHC, achieved using multiplex IHC and immunofluorescence (IF), was significantly better at predicting objective response to immune checkpoint inhibitors (ICIs)(免疫检查点抑制剂) compared with gene expression profiling (GEP) (基因表达谱分析)or IHC alone, indicating the need for more complex computational approaches to decipher the underlying biology and enhance clinical utility.

5. The development and integration of digital pathology and AI-based approaches provide substantive advantages over traditional methods, such as enabling spatial analysis while generating highly precise, unbiased, and consistent readouts that can be accessed remotely by pathologists.

6. Efforts to overcome some of the challenges seen with traditional pathology methods have led to the development and adoption of complex, novel imaging systems and whole slide image (WSI)(全视野数字切片)scanners that have enabled the transition of pathology into the digital era, also known as digital pathology. Within minutes, WSI scanners capture multiple images of entire tissue sections on the slide, which are digitally stitched together to generate a WSI that can be reviewed by a pathologist on a computer monitor. Two scanners, Philips IntelliSite Pathology Solution (PIPS) (Philips, Amsterdam, Netherlands) and Leica Aperio AT2 DX System (Leica Biosystems, Buffalo Grove, Illinois, USA), are approved by the FDA for review and interpretation of digital surgical pathology slides prepared from biopsied tissue.

7. There are many practical advantages to using these digital pathology image systems and solutions that would bring substantial benefits to translational and clinical research. These include the organization and storage of large amounts of data in a centralized location, integration of digital workflow software to help streamline

processes and improve efficiency, convenient sharing of image data to enable cross-specialty worldwide remote communication, reduced testing turnaround time, and the generation of precise and highly reproducible tissue-derived readouts reducing inter-pathologist variability. The increased speed and efficiency gained in image acquisition can enhance the downstream utilization options of traditional techniques such as hematoxylin and eosin (H&E)(苏木精和伊红), IHC, and in situ hybridization(杂交). These slides can be converted into a remotely available image within minutes and centrally reviewed by multiple pathologists from various sites, with applications including education, research, consultation, and diagnostics.

8. Recently, due to ongoing disruptions in relation to the COVID – 19 pandemic, including remote working and restricted travel, digital pathology has been crucial in the continuation of clinical and academic research, as well as routine pathology services. Without the need to transport glass slides and the ensuing logistical and safety concerns, central pathology review enables secure remote working. Additionally, the utilization of digital images allows the generation of pixel-level pattern information, leading to expanded use of computational approaches that enable a quantitative analysis of WSIs.

9. The use of digital image analysis in pathology can identify and quantify specific cell types quickly and accurately and can quantitatively evaluate histological features, morphological patterns, and biologically relevant regions of interest. Quantitative image analysis tools also enable the capturing of data from tissue slides that may not be accessible during manual assessment via routine microscopy. Additionally, performing similar tasks manually can require significant time investment and can be prone to human error, such as counting fatigue.

10. Quantitative image analysis can also be used to generate high-content data through application to a technique known as multiplexing, which allows co-expression and co-localization analysis of multiple markers in situ with respect to the complex spatial context of tissue regions, including the stroma(基质), tumor parenchyma, and invasive margin. Current imaging metrics can utilize multispectral unmixing strategies to reveal co-expression patterns that define unique cell phenotypes and spatial relationships.

11. Automated classification of epithelial and immune cells and simultaneous marker analysis at the single-cell level has been conducted using prostate cancer, pancreatic adenocarcinoma, and melanoma(黑素瘤) tissue samples. Application of this technique allowed identification of distinct T-cell populations and their spatial distributions and underscored the potential of immune markers to identify patients who may benefit from immunotherapy(免疫治疗).

12. While a highly multiplexed imaging platform can be used to understand intra- and inter-cellular signaling pathways by examining how phenotypically distinct cell

populations are spatially distributed relative to one another，it is a time-consuming process applicable to a predefined region of interest. However，as technology quickly advances，allowing digital evaluation of entire tissue slides，we are no longer confined to a region of interest. The wealth of new information provided by these techniques has created a need for more consistent and reproducible interpretation of large and complex datasets，along with defining the interaction patterns between cell types and spatial context found in pathological images（病理图像）that define biological underpinnings.

13. The need for data reproducibility and the increasing complexity of the analyses described above has led to the application of AI in pathology. AI refers to a broad scientific discipline that involves using algorithms to train machines to extract information or features beyond human visual perception. AI approaches are built to initially extract appropriate image representations and then to train a machine classifier for a particular segmentation，diagnostic，or prognostic task using a supervised or unsupervised approach. The power of AI to analyze large amounts of data quickly can significantly speed up the discovery of novel histopathology features that may aid our understanding of or ability to predict how a patient's disease will progress and how the patient will likely respond to a specific treatment. In breast cancer，for example，unsupervised learning models have been used to generate histologic scores that can differentiate between low-and high-grade tumors and evaluate prognostically relevant morphological features from the epithelium（上皮）and stroma of tissue samples to provide a score associated with the probability of overall survival. The success of these AI-based approaches relies on the quality and quantity of the data used to train the algorithm，limiting the generalizability of these image analysis algorithms to larger or more complex datasets.

From Modern Pathology，2022，35（1）

New words and expression

pathology /pə'θɒlədʒi/ *n*. the scientific study of diseases 病理学

mechanism /'mekənɪzəm/ *n*. a system of parts in a living thing that together perform a particular function（生物体内的）机制，构造

efficacy /'efɪkəsi/ *n*. the ability of sth，especially a drug or a medical treatment，to produce the results that are wanted（尤指药物或治疗方法的）功效，效验，效力

surrogate /'sʌrəgət/ *adj*. used to describe a person or thing that takes the place of，or is used instead of，sb/sth else 替代的；代用的

formalin /'fɔməlɪn/ *n*. a 10% solution of formaldehyde in water 甲醛（水溶）液；蚁醛；福尔马林

variability /ˌveərɪə'bɪləti/ *n*. the fact of sth being likely to vary 可变性；易变性；反复不定

identification /aɪˌdentɪfɪˈkeɪʃn/ *n*. the process of showing, proving or recognizing who or what sb/sth is 鉴定；辨认

integration /ˌɪntɪˈɡreɪʃn/ *n*. the act or process of combining two or more things so that they work together (= of integrating them) 结合；整合；一体化

pathologist /pəˈθɒlədʒɪst/ *n*. a doctor who studies pathology and examines dead bodies to find out the cause of death 病理学医生；病理学家

pandemic /pænˈdemɪk/ *n*. a disease that spreads over a whole country or the whole world （全国或全球性）流行病；大流行病

metastasis /məˈtæstəsɪs/ *n*. the development of tumours in different parts of the body resulting from cancer that has started in another part of the body （瘤）转移

toxicology /ˌtɒksɪˈkɒlədʒi/ *n*. the scientific study of poisons 毒理学；毒物学

After reading

Task 3　Read Text A again and answer the following questions.

1. What is the influence of Artificial Intelligence on pathology?

2. What are the practical advantages of using these digital pathology image systems and solutions that would bring substantial benefits to translational and clinical research?

Task 4　Check your vocabulary. Fill in the blanks with the correct form of the words from the following box, each word can be used only once.

> aggregate(*adj*.)　　fraternal(*adj*.)　　lens(*n*.)　　liable(*adj*.)　　nuclear(*adj*.)
> oxygen(*n*.)　pendulum(*n*.)　postulate(*v*.)　reproduce(*v*.)　subordinate(*adj*.)
> supreme(*adj*.)

1. Lesions in the cornea could be caused by physical damage (e.g., small particles in the air, plant matter) or by improper care for contact _____.

2. On the other hand, if the patient needs to be treated or moved around, I have to designate that chore to a specially trained doctor or nurse so that I would not be _____ in case of an accident or malpractice.

3. A contact at the school is important to set up an _____ for the presentation.

4. The five main concept designs were a _____, a drop impact tester, a rail gun, a coil gun, and a pneumatic gun.

5. What started as a single-protest against a factory later led residents to pursue action about truck traffic, argue their case at the _____ Court, and form a partnership with a local college.

6. While X-ray imaging is used for bony, dense structures, Magnetic Resonance

Imaging (MRI), an application of _____ Magnetic Resonance, has been used with soft tissues for decades.

7. We report the case of _____ twins presenting with severe hypochromic microcytic anemia and hypoferritinemia.

8. Additionally, during aggressive interactions between male adult rats, 22 kHz USVs have been recorded from _____ rats, which are thought to be an indication of submission in order to inhibit attacks from dominant rats.

9. These developing forests generated _____ as a photosynthetic waste product, thus increasing its abundance in the atmosphere and making the land a much more suitable place for animal life.

10. All bird species _____ through the use of a cleidoic egg, a structure which utilizes a hard shell to protect the developing embryo inside.

Task 5   Build your vocabulary. Read the sentences below, decide which word in each bracket is more suitable.

1. Finally it is plausible that some of these nations, particularly nations with large Muslim populations, may become strong United States (allies/friends), or at the very least no longer be enemies of the United States.

2. I hypothesized that the best quality journals would be most selective in accepting submissions and therefore would be most likely to publish articles which strongly (follow/adhere to) the scientific method.

3. This is shown in the (metaphor/simile) prosed by Simon of a building with several large rooms, each of which is divided up into cubicles.

4. Outbreaks in turkeys in North America, which (coincided/synchronised) with the fall migration of waterfowl, and serological surveys of asymptomatic pig farm workers were the only indicators of regular interspecific transmission.

5. Even after the death of Queen Victoria in 1901, Victorian ideals about morality, class and women's roles (invaded/pervaded) the nation's thinking, as evidenced throughout the works of Brittain, Robert Roberts, and E.M. Forster. However, kernels of change—expansion of political activity, education and the role of government—had arisen in the late nineteenth century.

6. Though their satisfactions to the performance of his government, especially in regard to economic growth, the majority of Thai people are still (reluctant/unhappy) to accept GMOs and could potentially reflect their discontent in the coming election.

7. On the other hand, the difference in the values for the rigor (contents/index) is more likely to reflect an actual disparity between the ways in which ecological research is framed at the two institutions.

8. Yet, this is not a simple task. The fact that typical financial impediments such as

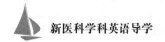

lower academic achievement and unemployment were associated with suicide attempts speaks to the intersectionality of social factors that may contribute to the (detriment/expense) of mental health.

9. We have learnt in the chapter on Money and Inflation that this complaint about inflation reducing the purchasing power of labor is a common (error/fallacy).

10. Frog Island Community Garden is one link in a network of community gardens in Ypsilanti that are working to combat this (trend/pattern) of unhealthy eating.

Guiding to learn

Task 6   Learn the following general academic vocabulary.

consistently community consequently normal textual considerable conventional demonstrate framework outcome sequence approximately dimension grant status alter evolution acknowledge aggregation diverse exceed underlying comprehensively comprise empirical innovative accumulation biased infrastructure intensive bulk format unify

Beginning to read

Task 7   Now read the text.

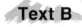

Big Data in Basic and Translational Cancer Research

Peng Jiang & Eytan Ruppin et al

1. Cancer is a complex process, and its progression involves diverse processes in the patient's body. Consequently, the cancer research community generates massive amounts of molecular and phenotypic（表型的） data to study cancer hallmarks as comprehensively as possible. The rapid accumulation of omics data catalysed by breakthroughs in high-throughput technologies has given rise to the notion of "big data" in cancer, which we define as a dataset with two basic properties: first, it contains abundant information that can give novel insights into essential questions, and

second，its analysis demands a large computer infrastructure beyond equipment available to an individual researcher—an evolving concept as computational resources evolve exponentially following Moore's law. A model example of such big data is the dataset collected by The Cancer Genome Atlas（TCGA）（癌症基因组图谱）. TCGA contains 2.5 petabytes of raw data—an amount 2,500 times greater than modern laptop storage in 2022—and requires specialized computers for storage and analysis. Further，between its initial release in 2008 to March 2022，at least 10,242 articles and 11,054 NIH（美国国家卫生研究院）grants cited TCGA according to a PubMed search，demonstrating its transformative value as a community resource that has markedly driven cancer research forward.

2. Big data are not unique to the cancer field，and play an essential role in many scientific disciplines，notably cosmology，weather forecasting and image recognition. However，datasets in the cancer field differ from those in other fields in several key aspects. First，the size of cancer datasets is typically markedly smaller. For example，in March 2022，the US National Center for Biotechnology Information（NCBI）（国家生物技术信息中心）Gene Expression Omnibus（GEO）（基因表达综合数据库）database—the largest genomics data repository to our knowledge—contained approximately 1.1 million samples with "cancer" as a keyword. However，ImageNet，the largest public repository for computer vision，contains 15 million images. Second，cancer research data are typically heterogeneous and may contain many dimensions measuring distinct aspects of cellular systems and biological processes. Modern multi-omics workflows may generate genome-wide mRNA（信使核糖核酸）expression，chromatin accessibility and protein expression data on single cells，together with a spatial molecular readout. The comparatively limited data size in each modality and the high heterogeneity among them necessitate the development of innovative computational approaches for integrating data from different dimensions and cohorts.

3. The subject of big data in cancer is of immense scope，and it is impossible to cover everything in one review. We therefore focus on key big-data analyses that led to conceptual advances in our understanding of cancer biology and impacted disease diagnosis（诊断）and treatment decisions. Further，we detail reviews in the pertaining sections to direct interested readers to relevant resources. We acknowledge that our limited selection of topics and examples may omit important work，for which we sincerely apologize.

4. In this Review，we begin by describing major data sources. Next，we review and discuss data analysis approaches designed to leverage big datasets for cancer discoveries. We then introduce ongoing efforts to harness big data in clinically oriented，translational studies，the primary focus of this Review. Finally，we discuss current challenges and future steps to push forward big data use in cancer.

5. There are five basic data types in cancer research：molecular omics data，

perturbation phenotypic data，molecular（分子）interaction data，imaging data，and textual data. Molecular omics data describe the abundance or status of molecules in cellular systems and tissue samples. Such data are the most abundant type generated in cancer research from patient or preclinical samples，and include information on DNA（脱氧核糖核酸）mutations chromatin or DNA states，protein abundance，transcript abundance and metabolite abundance. Early studies relied on data from bulk samples to provide insights into cancer progressions，tumour heterogeneity and tumour evolution，by using well-designed computational approaches. Following the development of single-cell technologies and decreases in sequencing costs，current molecular data can be generated at multi sample and single-cell levels and reveal tumour heterogeneity and evolution at a much higher resolution. Furthermore，genomic and transcriptomic readouts can include spatial information，revealing cancer clonal（无性繁殖系的）evolutions within distinct regions and gene expression changes associated with clone-specific aberrations（像差）.

6. Perturbation phenotypic data describe how cell phenotypes，such as cell proliferation or the abundance of marker proteins，are altered following the suppression or amplification of gene levels or drug treatments. Common phenotyping experiments include perturbation screens using CRISPR（规律间隔成簇短回文重复序列）knockout，interference or activation；RNA（核糖核酸）interference；overexpression of open reading frames；or treatment with a library of drugs. As a limitation，the generation of perturbation phenotypic data from clinical samples is still challenging due to the requirement of genetically manipulable live cells.

7. Molecular interaction data describe the potential function of molecules through their interacting with diverse partners. Common molecular interaction data types include data on protein-DNA interactions，protein-RNA interactions，protein-protein interactions and 3D chromosomal interactions. Similar to perturbation phenotypic data，molecular interaction data sets（数据集）are typically generated using cell lines as their generation requires a large quantity of material that often exceeds that available from clinical samples.

8. Clinical data such as health records，histopathology（组织病理学）images and radiology（放射学）images can also be of considerable value. The boundary between molecular omics and image data is not absolute as both can include information of the other type，for example in datasets that contain imaging scans and information on protein expression from a tumour sample.

9. We provide an overview of key data resources for cancer research organized in three categories. The first category comprises resources from projects that systematically generate data；for example，TCGA generated transcriptomic，proteomic，genomic and epigenomic data for more than 10,000 cancer genomes and matched normal samples，spanning 33 cancer types. The second category describes

repositories presenting processed data from the aforementioned projects，such as the Genomic Data Commons(基因组数据共享)，which hosts TCGA data for downloading. The third category includes Web applications that systematically integrate data across diverse projects and provide interactive analysis modules. For example，the TIDE(肿瘤免疫功能障碍和排斥)framework systematically collected public data from immuno-oncology studies and provided interactive modules to study pathways and regulation mechanisms underlying tumour immune evasion and immunotherapy response.

10. In addition to cancer-focused large-scale projects enumerated in Table 2，many individual groups have deposited genomic(染色体组的)datasets that are useful for cancer research in general databases such as GEO3 and Array Express. Curation of these datasets could lead to new resources for cancer biology studies. For example，the PRECOG database contains 166 transcriptomic studies collected from GEO and Array Express with patient survival information for querying the association between gene expression and prognostic outcome.

11. Although data-intensive studies may generate omics data on hundreds of patients，the data scale in cancer research is still far behind that in other fields，such as computer vision. Cross-cohort(跨队列)aggregation and cross-modality(跨模态)integration can markedly enhance the robustness and depth of big data analysis. We discuss these strategies in the following subsections.

12. Cross-cohort data aggregation. Integration of datasets from multiple centres or studies can achieve more robust results and potentially new findings，especially where individual datasets are noisy，incomplete or biased with certain artefacts. A landmark of cross-cohort data aggregation is the discovery of the TMPRSS2–ERG fusion and a less frequent TMPRSS2–ETV1 fusion as oncogenic drivers in prostate cancer. A compendium analysis across 132 gene-expression datasets representing 10，486 microarray(微阵列)experiments first identified ERG and ETV1 as highly expressed genes in six independent prostate(前列腺)cancer cohorts32，further studies identified their fusions with TMPRSS2 as the cause of ERG and ETV1 over-expression.

13. A general approach for cross-cohort aggregation is to obtain public datasets that are related to a new research topic or have similar study designs to a new dataset. However，use of public data for a new analysis is challenging because the experimental design behind each published dataset is unique，requiring labour-intensive expert interpretation and manual standardization. A recent framework for data curation provides natural language processing and semi-automatic functions to unify datasets with heterogeneous meta-information into a format usable for algorithmic(算法的)analysis.

14. Although data aggregation may generate robust hypotheses，batch effects caused by differences in laboratories，individual researcher's techniques or platforms or other non-biological factors may mask or reduce the strength of signals uncovered，

and correcting for these effects is therefore a critical step in cross-cohort aggregations
（聚集体）. Popular batch effect correction approaches include the ComBat package，
which uses empirical Bayes estimators to compute corrected data，and the Seurat
package，which creates integrated single-cell clusters（簇）anchored on similar cells
between batches.

From Nature Reviews Cancer，*2022*，*22: 625 − 639*

After reading

Task 8 Build your vocabulary.

Directions： Match the following words with their corresponding definitions and
Chinese equivalents.

English： phenotypic repository heterogeneous heterogeneity computational
perturbation cellular metabolite

Chinese： 表型的 贮藏室 成分混杂的 异质性 与计算机有关的 小变异 细胞的
代谢物

Paras. 1—7

English	Chinese	Definition
1. _____	_____	a. of or relating to or constituting a phenotype
2. _____	_____	b. a place where sth is stored in large quantities
3. _____	_____	c. consisting of many different kinds of people or things
4. _____	_____	d. the quality of being diverse and not comparable in kind
5. _____	_____	e. using or connected with computers
6. _____	_____	f. a small change in the quality，behaviour or movement of sth
7. _____	_____	g. connected with or consisting of the cells of plants or animals
8. _____	_____	h. any substance involved in metabolism（either as a product of metabolism or as necessary for metabolism）

Paras. 8—14

English: radiology　aforementioned　immunotherapy　enumerate　prognostic　compendium　dysfunction

Chinese: 放射学　上述的　免疫疗法　列举　预兆的　摘要　机能障碍

English	Chinese	Definition
9. _____	_____	i. the study and use of different types of radiation in medicine，for example to treat diseases
10. _____	_____	j. mentioned before，in an earlier sentence
11. _____	_____	k. therapy designed to produce immunity to a disease or to enhance resistance by the immune system
12. _____	_____	l. to name things on a list one by one
13. _____	_____	m. of or relating to prediction
14. _____	_____	n. a collection of facts，drawings and photographs on a particular subject，especially in a book
15. _____	_____	o. If someone has a physical dysfunction，part of their body is not working properly.

Guiding to learn

Task 9　Learn the following general academic vocabulary from the word bank.

accompany available insight differentiating evaluate intelligence integrate dimensional extraction facilitate emerging validation dramatically ultimately concentration variations automated subsequent capability

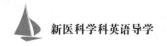

Beginning to read

Task 10　Now read the text.

Text C

Proteomic Profiling and Artificial Intelligence for Hepatocellular Carcinoma Translational Medicine

Nurbubu T. Moldogazieva et al

1. Hepatocellular carcinoma（HCC）（肝细胞癌）is a multifactorial heterogeneous disease and the most common primary malignant tumor of the liver with increasing incidence rate worldwide. HCC is the fifth diagnosed cancer and the second most frequent cause of cancer-related deaths in men and the ninth cancer case and the sixth cause of deaths from cancers in women. Liver cirrhosis（肝硬化）is a main cause of HCC and together with inflammation associated with hepatitis B virus（HBV）（乙型肝炎病毒）or hepatitis C virus（HCV）（丙型肝炎病毒）accompanies early stages of HCC. Consequently，diagnostic and prognostic biomarkers with high specificity and sensitivity for HCC diagnosis at an early stage and differentiation between HCC and non-diseases are of crucial importance. Moreover，monitoring patient's postoperative status and treatment efficacy along with evaluation of disease progression and metastasis risk to predict cancer recurrence are needed.

2. HCC is typically diagnosed by liver biopsy or cross-sectional liver imaging techniques such as contrast-enhanced computer tomography（CT）（电子计算机断层扫描）and magnetic resonance imaging（MRI）（磁共振成像）. These techniques are useful for tumor staging and detecting extrahepatic metastases，which involve，mostly，lungs，lymph nodes，bone，adrenal glands，and peritoneum. Usage imaging criteria according to Liver Imaging Reporting and Data System（LI-RADS）（肝脏影像报告和数据系统）and introduction of novel imaging technologies such as contrast-enhanced liver ultrasound can improve early diagnosis and differentiating HCC from non-HCC liver diseases to increase surveillance of HCC patients. However，some limitations in imaging approaches such as time consuming and low sensitivity dictate necessity of developing both novel screening methods and highly sensitive and specific biomarkers for HCC early diagnosis and prognosis.

3. Currently available integrative genomic/epigenomic/transcriptomic/proteomic profiling approaches and biomarker assay techniques provide multifaceted insight into

biomarker discovery. Comprehensive multiomics profiling enables differentiating early and advanced HCCs as well as HCC from chronic liver diseases, even without knowledge of the clinical symptoms. Additionally, this allows assessing intra-tumoral phenotypic heterogeneity(肿瘤内表型异质性) and uncovering individual variability and alterations in unique gene expression patterns, which underlie tumor initiation and progression. Multiomics-based platforms are used for molecular classification of HCC subtypes characterized by different driver genes to provide deeper insight into cancer pathogenesis and to evaluate the potency of genomic, epigenomic, and proteomic signatures as HCC biomarkers.

4. The challenge in multiomics technologies is the accumulation of a huge amount of very heterogeneous raw data stored in different data formats. A large amount of complex heterogeneous data is referred to as big data, which are described by top "V's" characteristics such as value, volume, velocity, variety, veracity, and variability. Big data analytics in cancer implies the integration, analysis, interpretation, validation, and quality control of large datasets from thousands of patients. This requires suitable and promising open-source distributed data processing software platforms.

5. Significant progress has been achieved due to the application of artificial intelligence (AI) technologies, which enhance healthcare data collection and interpretation. This is provided by computer-based algorithms for data analysis and by the construction of predictive models for improving image recognition and representation in HCC diagnosis and prognosis. Additionally, AI arises as a powerful tool in the analysis and integration of complex and heterogeneous datasets obtained due to multiomics profiling for disease staging, prediction of disease recurrence, monitoring treatment response, and the identification of diagnostic, prognostic, and predictive biomarkers.

6. Proteomics(蛋白质组学) is a large-scale investigation and analysis of proteins aimed to identify and characterizing proteomes as a complete protein composition of a cell or tissue. Proteomics implies protein distribution profiling and protein expression/ activity patterning and protein-protein interaction identification. Current integrated proteomic profiling technologies use hybrid platforms based on multi-dimensional (MD) separations and three-dimensional (3D) liquid chromatography (LC)(液相色谱) and have provided powerful solutions. Currently available proteomic data from MS-based proteomic experiments are integrated in public repositories such as ProteomeXchange Consortium, Proteomics Identification (PRIDE), Human Plasma Peptide Atlas. These repositories provide efficient and reliable dissemination, comparative analysis, interpretation, and extraction of proteomic data.

7. Translational medicine implies, on the one hand, application of new knowledge into clinical practice to increase efficacy of a disease diagnosis and therapeutic

strategies and，on the other hand，to facilitate generation of new hypotheses from clinical observations. The aim of translational medicine is combination of benchside，bedside and community in the enhancement of patient's care decision making. Integrated data from diverse omics technologies enable the large-scale identification of novel molecular biomarkers for translating them into clinical practice. Thus，translating knowledge on a biomarker structure，functions，and expression into clinical practice should enable HCC early diagnosis，prognosis，and assessment of treatment efficacy. However，limited success has been achieved in translating cancer biomarker proteomic profiling（癌症生物标志物蛋白质组学分析）into clinical practice.

8. Our review focuses on the recent advancements in the integrative proteomic profiling strategies and emerging AI technologies for discovery of novel biomarkers for HCC early diagnosis and prognosis. We discuss proteomic signatures of HCC，starting from conventional and promising biomarkers and alterations in cell signaling pathways involved in hepatocarcinogenesis（肝癌形成）. This is followed by consideration of the latest findings in exploring novel proteomic biomarker candidates with emphasis on their translational application.

From Biomedicines，*2021*，*9（159）*

New words and expressions

malignant /mə'lɪɡnənt/ *adj*. that cannot be controlled and is likely to cause death（of a tumour or disease）恶性的

hepatitis /ˌhepə'taɪtɪs/ *n*. a serious disease of the liver. There are three main forms：hepatitis A（the least serious，caused by infected food），hepatitis B and hepatitis C（both very serious and caused by infected blood）肝炎

prognosis /prɒɡ'nəʊsɪs/ *n*. an opinion，based on medical experience，of the likely development of a disease or an illness（对病情的）预断，预后

variability /ˌveərɪə'bɪləti/ *n*. the fact of sth being likely to vary 可变性；易变性；反复不定

molecular /mə'lekjələ(r)/ *adj*. relating to or involving molecules. 分子的

velocity /və'lɒsəti/ *n*. the speed of sth in a particular direction（沿某一方向的）速度

veracity /və'ræsəti/ *n*. the quality of being true 真实；真实性

algorithms /'ælɡərɪðəmz/ *n*. a series of mathematical steps，especially in a computer program，which will give you the answer to a particular kind of problem or question.（尤指电脑程序中的）算法；运算法则

dissemination /dɪˌsemɪ'neɪʃn/ *n*. the act of dispersing or diffusing something 传播；宣传；散播；传染（病毒）

tomography /tə'mɒɡrəfi/ *n*. a way of producing an image of the inside of the human body or a solid object using X-rays or ultrasound 体层摄影（利用 X 射线和超声波清楚显示体内结构）

After reading

Task 11   Build your vocabulary. Choose one word which can be used to replace the language shown in bold without changing the meaning of the sentence from the list below. Change forms and cases when necessary.

| allude(v.)   cater (v.)   discern (v.)   drug (n.)   evolve (v.)   launch (v.) |
| proclaim(v.)   rebel(n.)   territory(n.)   testify(v.)   utilise(n.) |

1. It is now assumed that limbs with digits **developed gradually** completely for aquatic adaptation.   _____

2. He has **announced** the island to be his own; he repeatedly refers to places on the island as his, showcasing his inherently possessive nature.   _____

3. The problem is not that the government completely ignores the food system and the crisis of diet related illness, but rather that the government comes up with solutions that **provide** too much to the food lobbies.   _____

4. We also participate in ethnocentrism when we insist that the post-colony survivor **give evidence** to re-integrate traumatic memory and achieve psychic coherence.

   _____

5. Treatment presents its own problems; large doses of **medicines** may cause sudden destruction of many bacteria, which would then release large amounts of toxin into the bloodstream, hastening death.   _____

6. I will **make use of** the same GeneChip for the Arabidopsis genome as used by Paul et al. in their experiment.   _____

7. The austere approach to the design is almost difficult to **notice** from the modernistic design. But I believe I see it in the entrance to the Grove of Meditation.

   _____

8. Floaters are individuals that have not established a **space**, so they do not breed, even though they may be old enough to reproduce.   _____

9. We don't know exactly what was produced on the Redlund farm, but information from the region and information about Hjalmer do **refer** to a story.

   _____

10. We **initiate** invasive removal projects to save the natives; however, are we actually helping them by removing an invasive?   _____

Further reading

Baxi, V., Edwards, R., Montalto, M., et al. (2022). Digital Pathology and Artificial Intelligence in Translational Medicine and Clinical Practice. *Modern Pathology*.

35(1).

Bernstam，E. V.，Shireman，P. K.，Meric-Bernstam，F.，et al.（2022）. Artificial Intelligence in Clinical and Translational Science：Successes，Challenges and Opportunities. *Clinical and Translational Science*. 15(2).

Ding，L.，Bradford，C.，Kuo，I. L.，et al.（2022）. Radiation Oncology：Future Vision for Quality Assurance and Data Management in Clinical Trials and Translational Science. *Frontiers in Oncology*. 12(8).

Jiang，P.，Sinha，S.，Aldape，K.，et al.（2022）. Big Data in Basic and Translational Cancer Research. *Nature Reviews Cancer*. 22(11).

Moldogazieva，N. T.，Mokhosoev，I. M.，Zavadskiy，S. P.，et al.（2021）. Proteomic Profiling and Artificial Intelligence for Hepatocellular Carcinoma Translational Medicine. *Biomedicines*. 9(2).

Unit 9
Artificial Intelligence in Medical Diagnosis

Guiding to learn

Advances in Artificial Intelligence (AI), particularly in deep learning, have made it possible to extract clinically relevant information from complex and diverse clinical datasets. It also provides researchers with unprecedented possibilities for dynamic and complex biological genomic analyses. What's more, AI can be of tremendous help in analyzing raw image data from cardiac imaging techniques (such as echocardiography, computed tomography, cardiac MRI among others) and electrocardiogram recordings through incorporation of an algorithm.

Discuss the following questions with your partners.

1. What are the disadvantages of classical machine learning techniques?
2. What is the value of genetic testing gap in cardiovascular diseases?
3. What is the difference between classification of learning and deep learning?

Task 1 **Learn the following general academic vocabulary.**

assessment available conceptually interpretation procedure process specifically complex computational consequently normally primarily regulatory dominate validation adequately emerging implementation parameter subsequently external facilities generate flexible interval definitive publication ambiguity automate detection guideline infrastructure intensity prospective random supplementary assemble

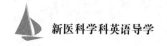

Beginning to read

Task 2   Now read the text.

Text A

Artificial Intelligence in Liver Diseases: Improving Diagnostics, Prognostics and Response Prediction
David Nam et al

Hepatology—a complex art

1. Hepatology（肝脏病学）is the clinical study of liver disease and is a prime example of the complexity of modern medicine. To diagnose disease, make a prognosis about disease outcomes, and recommend an optimal treatment, clinicians rely on a vast array of diagnostic data modalities. The standard clinical workup of patients with suspected or confirmed liver disease includes taking the clinical history, performing a clinical examination, running laboratory tests, and interpreting imaging studies. Liver biopsies（活组织检查）may even be performed, requiring assessment of changes in tissues, cells and molecular markers. Collectively, these data modalities contain a wealth of information. Interpretation of this information is a challenging task, even for seasoned clinicians, and diagnostic ambiguities abound in hepatology.

Machine learning and deep learning

2. Artificial intelligence (AI) enables computers to learn from complex datasets and solve real-world problems within and beyond medicine, leading to performances on par with or better than those of their human counterparts. AI refers to computational approaches to data analysis in which computer programs are not explicitly guided by experts but primarily learn from examples. Throughout this article, we will use AI as a broad term that includes classical machine learning (ML)（机器语言）and deep learning (DL)（深度学习）techniques. Classical ML techniques do not require dedicated hardware and have been used for decades in medicine, including hepatology and gastroenterology（胃肠病学）studies. These techniques rely on "handcrafted features" defined by human investigators. What does this mean in the context of hepatology? An example of AI as applied to hepatology is automatic prognostication of solid tumors based on imaging data. Using a handcrafted approach,

human investigators assemble a list of quantitative visual features such as tumour size, roundness, symmetry and intensity on images. These features are subsequently inputted into a classification algorithm, for example, the "random forest" method, which excels at categorizing such tabular data. In radiology（放射学）image analysis, handcrafted image analysis approaches are traditionally termed "radiomics"（or "classical radiomics"）. In addition to this established ML approach, "deep learning"（DL）has blossomed in the last 10 years thanks to algorithmic advances, improved hardware, and large datasets. While conceptually similar to classical ML approaches, DL methods usually have thousands more free parameters than classical ML methods. This abundance of parameters makes DL models more flexible and better suited for processing and classifying complex data sets such as language data or imaging data. In medicine, the most commonly used DL methods are artificial neural networks（used for image processing and processing of time series）and transformers（used for language processing and, more recently, image processing）. Importantly, in a DL approach, investigators do not assemble lists of handcrafted features. Rather, a DL network is entrusted with automatically finding features associated with an endpoint, specifically the clinical outcome. Given today's technologies, DL methods usually outperform handcrafted feature-based approaches and consequently dominate the field of AI in hepatology. However, the demarcation（划界）between handcrafted approaches and DL is not absolute; multiple studies have used DL systems to extract features, which are subsequently combined with handcrafted features. Application-wise, ML/DL approaches can be used for two ends. First, they can recapitulate, and thus automate, the interpretation of data normally performed by human experts. Second, they can extract subtle features from complex data which are not immediately obvious to the human eye.

Academic research on AI in hepatology

3. Academic research groups from multiple countries are actively engaged in ML/DL research in hepatology. Based on a quantitative survey of the MEDLINE database, researchers from China and the USA are the most prolific, with between 30 and 40 total publications on ML/DL in hepatology. By far the most common application is automatic diagnosis of liver disease from imaging data. In these cases, the ground truth is derived from the image data itself. For instance, an expert radiologist diagnoses a malignant liver mass in a CT（计算机断层扫描）data set and the ML/DL algorithm is tasked with reproducing this diagnosis in a supervised training experiment. Another group of studies involves prognosis prediction from image-based data. Forecasting the natural course of a disease can have direct implications for the clinical management of patients. Accurate prognostication allows clinicians to adjust follow-up intervals, convey the urgency of lifestyle changes to patients, and adjust the intensity or type of

pharmacological treatment. A third category of applications is segmentation of structures of interest. Segmentation studies aim to generate an accurate outline around a region of interest. As a clinical example, algorithms can delineate organs at risk before radiation therapy of cancer. While ML/DL studies in hepatology address a range of diseases, almost all published studies address either neoplastic or metabolic diseases of the liver, which are the major causes of liver-related morbidity and mortality besides viral hepatitis. ML/DL studies in hepatology currently incorporate a range of imaging modalities. The 3 most commonly analyzed modalities are CT scans, MRI(核磁共振成像) scans and H&E-stained histopathology(组织病理学) slides. In the last 4 years, the number of ML/DL studies in hepatology has exponentially grown, even more so in radiology than in histopathology, and only 1 study has combined both data modalities so far. In addition, a trend toward a larger growth of DL studies compared to handcrafted feature-based studies can be observed.

Implementation of AI in hepatology

4. At this point, a number of ML/DL tools are already approved for clinical use by the US FDA(食品及药物管理局) and similar regulatory agencies worldwide. Nevertheless, there is a wide gap between the burgeoning number of research articles and the limited number of clinically approved, available applications. This discrepancy is exacerbated by missing external and prospective validation of models, lack of technological infrastructure in health facilities, lack of knowledge and trust in ML/DL systems among medical personnel, as well as data privacy issues. Furthermore, the clinical implementation of ML and DL methods in hepatology lags far behind that in other fields of medicine. Recently, the first ML/DL algorithms for management of patients with liver diseases were clinically approved in Europe and the US. In contrast, ML/DL algorithms have already been available in other areas of medicine for a few years, such as polyp(息肉) detection in colonoscopy(结肠镜检查), fracture detection in X-ray images and brain volume quantification in magnetic resonance scans. This is possibly due to the complex nature of hepatology, which rarely depends on a single data type for diagnosis and clinical management. In the following sections, we will review the current progress of ML/DL in hepatology from clinical and technical perspectives, focusing on histopathology and radiology image analysis.

AI in liver histopathology

5. One of the key challenges in liver histopathology is the clinical decision to obtain liver tissue via biopsy. While liver biopsy is a safe procedure for most patients, it is associated with non-negligible morbidity(不可忽略发病率). Moreover, national guidelines and clinical practice are not always consistent about when a biopsy's benefits

outweigh its risks. This explains the obvious need for noninvasive biomarkers and likely explains the abundance of ML/DL studies in liver radiology. Nevertheless，once a biopsy has been obtained，there is a clinical need for a fast，definitive，reliable，reproducible and quantitative diagnosis. It was not until 2020 that the application of ML/DL methods in liver histopathology gathered pace. Unlike radiology which adopted radiomics in several studies，histopathology did not extensively apply ML methods using handcrafted features. Rather，most research groups immediately adopted emerging DL algorithms based on convolutional neural networks（CNNs）（卷积神经网络），which were originally developed for non-medical computer vision tasks.

6. Most studies in histopathology have used data from patients with non-alcoholic fatty liver disease（NAFLD）（非酒精性脂肪肝病），non-alcoholic steatohepatitis（NASH）（非酒精性脂肪性肝炎）or hepatocellular carcinoma（HCC）（肝细胞癌）. All of these diseases share the clinical need for clear-cut diagnostic and prognostic systems. Several studies have focused on models quantifying steatosis，inflammation，hepatocellular ballooning and other morphological patterns in patients with NAFLD，as well as the staging of liver fibrosis. In 2014，Vanderbeck et al. published one of the first studies using handcrafted features in a support vector machine algorithm to identify and quantify macrosteatosis（大泡性脂肪变），central veins，bile ducts and other structures on scanned H&E slides from NAFLD and healthy liver biopsies，with an overall accuracy of 89%. In the following year，the same group extended their algorithm for the classification of lobular inflammation and hepatocyte ballooning with AUCs of 0.95 and 0.98，respectively. Another study developed a ML quantifier of morphological features of NAFLD to calculate a diagnostic score for NASH，yielding an AUC of 0.80（95% CI 0.68－0.89）.

From JHEP Reports，*2022*，*4（4）*

New words and expressions

hepatology /ˌhɛpəˈtɒlədʒi/ *n*. the branch of medicine concerned with the liver and its diseases 肝脏病学；肝胆科

prognosis /prɒɡˈnəʊsɪs/ *n*. an opinion，based on medical experience，of the likely development of a disease or an illness（对病情的）预断，预后

counterpart /ˈkaʊntəpɑːt/ *n*. a person or thing that has the same position or function as sb/sth else in a different place or situation 职位（或作用）相当的人；对应的事物；配对物

explicitly /ɪksˈplɪsɪtli/ *adv*. Something that is explicit is expressed or shown clearly and openly，without any attempt to hide anything. 明确的；清晰的；毫不隐讳的

gastroenterology /ˌɡæstrəʊˌentərˈɒlədʒi/ *n*. the branch of medicine that studies the gastrointestinal tract and its diseases 胃肠病学；胃肠科

parameter /pəˈræmɪtə(r)/ *n*. something that decides or limits the way in which sth can be done 决定因素;规范;范围

transformer /trænsˈfɔːmə(r)/ *n*. a device for reducing or increasing the voltage of an electric power supply, usually to allow a particular piece of electrical equipment to be used 变压器;转换器

prolific /prəˈlɪfɪk/ *adj*. existing in large numbers or producing a Cot of fruit flowers, young 众多的;大批的;多产的;多育的

pharmacological /ˌfɑːməkəˈlɒdʒɪkəl/ *adj*. of or relating to pharmacology 药理学的

segmentation /ˌseɡmenˈteɪʃn/ *n*. the act of dividing sth into different parts; one of these parts 分割;划分

exponentially /ˌɛkspəˈnɛnʃ(ə)li/ *adv*. growing or increasing very rapidly 以指数方式;指数地

validation /ˌvælɪˈdeɪʃən/ *n*. the cognitive process of establishing a valid proof 确认;证实;核实

colonoscopy /ˌkəʊləˈnɒskəpi/ *n*. visual examination of the colon (with a colonoscope) from the cecum to the rectum 结肠镜检查

radiology /ˌreɪdiˈɒlədʒi/ *n*. the study and use of different types of radiation in medicine, for example to treat diseases 放射学;放射医疗

After reading

Task 3 Scan the text A again and answer the following questions.

1. What does "handcrafted features" mean in the context of hepatology?

2. What is the difference between "deep learning"（DL）and classical machine learning（ML）approaches?

3. What are the challenges in liver histopathology?

Task 4 Check your vocabulary. Fill in the blanks with the correct form of the words from the following box, each word can be used only once.

acid(*n*.)	battery(*n*.)	breed(*v*.)	carbon(*n*.)	illuminate(*v*.)	integer(*n*.)
lustre(*n*.)	matrix(*n*.)	molecule(*n*.)	prince(*n*.)	stationary(*adj*.)	

1. Physicochemical properties, physiological roles, and distribution in a human body Cholesterol is a lipid composed of a four-ring system flanked by a hydroxyl group at _____ 3 of the ring A and a branched hydro-carbon side chain at carbon 17 of the ring D.

2. Aspiration pneumonia after chemoxA8Cintensity-modulated radiation therapy of oropharyngeal carcinoma and its clinical and dysphagia-related predictors Klaudia

U. Hunter, _____ , MD, 5 Scott A. McLean, MD, 5 Gregory T.

3. Because the number of providers is a/an _____ and may exceed 2.

4. We further discriminate the bluster from the _____ by identifying the key challenges that AI has been shown to address, balanced with the potential issues with its usage, and the key requisites for its success.

5. Signatures are computed from derived classes in an unsupervised mode. Computational _____ phenotyping: A method of pheno-typing cells using quantitative multichannel molecular imaging, measured molecule concentrations as data vectors, and unsupervised classification of the molecular N-space.

6. However, Figure 3, E was created on the following assumption: in a paired uterine horn and cervix from 1 animal, the ratio of smooth muscle in each organ is relatively equal to that ratio in other animals of the same _____ , age, weight, and progress into pregnancy (ie, virgin, day 11, day 20).

7. Resolution of many autistic syndromes with respect to the relative contribution of specific genetic variants also continues to _____ understanding of the biology of autism comorbidities, such as ADHD, motor coordination impairment, epilepsy, intellectual disability, anxiety, and the psychopathologies.

8. Ogai *et al* evaluated physically active university students who performed the same protocol through strenuous workout on a/an _____ bike in two sessions.

9. Neurocognitive assessment details of neurocognitive _____ for each cohort are provided in the Supplementary Materials.

10. The single nucleotide polymorphism A118G codes for an amino _____ substitution Asp to Asn at the codon 40 and it is the most widely studied genetic variant of OPRM1.

Task 5 Build your vocabulary. Read the sentences below, decide which word in each bracket is more suitable.

1. Contributors The CFAS management committee all contributed to all aspects of the study, including (fund/finance) raising, design, supervision, and drafting.

2. Self-paced exercise offers an interesting test of this question, as the ability to modulate exercise intensity would theoretically permit the athlete to (tire/exhaust) the available muscular reserve to maximize performance and attain such a threshold of muscle fatigue.

3. The metamorphosis of the ideal woman follows the shifting role of women in society from mother and (girl friend/mistress) to a career-orientated individual.

4. While this expansion may be largely explained by general punishment trends, there appear to be unique factors that have prevented other (penal/punishment) reforms from similarly modulating sex offender punishment.

5. All other tissues exhibit much lower activities after 48 h with the exception of

bone, which displays uptake values of approximately 10 %ID/g, a consequence of the mineralization of (emancipated/liberated) 89Zr4 + in bone (Supplemental Fig. 22; Supplemental Tables 12 and 13).

6. The known biological effects of these metabolites suggest that alone or in combination, they could (evoke/provoke) retinal degeneration.

7. Overall, although they (divide/diverge) on subgroup analyses, the four trials report consistent data that bevacizumab could increase pathological complete response in patients with early breast cancer.

8. I shall hardly be induced to make any further trials of this kind because of the (torture/torment) of the creature but certainly the inquiry would be very noble if we could any way find a way soe to stupify the creature as that it might not be sensible which I fear there is hardly any opiate will performe.

9. This may be due to the (integral/intrinsic) limitations of extrapolating the results obtained from animal models to humans; however, as mentioned earlier, the most important limitation in humans is the definition of the phenotypes of aging.

10. If, as hypothesized, a particular variable represents a x810x899x810x810x810x834rate of change' of health, then its (accumulated/collected) history will be more predictive of mortality than its current single time value.

Guiding to learn

Task 6   Learn the following general academic vocabulary.

available consistent methodology procedure significant variant appropriate computational consequence impact inappropriate relevance circumstance component validation dimensional implementation statistical alteration facilitation fundamentally margin accuracy initiate utilize comprehensive confirmation definitive inference insertion automated conversely inherently revolutionized rigidly panel straightforward

Beginning to read

Task 7   Now read the text.

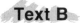

Text B

Artificial Intelligence and Cardiovascular Genetics
Chayakrit Krittanawong et al

1. Multiple diseases of the cardiovascular system are associated with genetic polymorphisms including both common conditions, such as hypercholesterolemia and less common conditions, such as cardiac channelopathies, cardiomyopathies, aortopathies, and various structural and congenital diseases of the heart and great vessels. Given that the fields of cardiovascular genetics and precision medicine are rapidly evolving, it is unsurprising that recently published guidelines include an increased focus on genetic testing. The 2020 Scientific Statement From the American Heart Association（AHA）（美国心脏协会）on Genetic Testing for Inherited Cardiovascular Diseases（遗传性心血管疾病）recommended testing specific genes in certain monogenic cardiovascular diseases（CVDs）in appropriate clinical circumstances The 2021 Scientific Statement from the AHA on Genetic Testing for Heritable Cardiovascular Diseases in Pediatric Patients also recommended cardiovascular genetic testing in children as an important component in determining the risk of developing heritable cardiovascular diseases in adulthood. With advancements in technology, several recent genetic studies have revealed potential targets for CVD screening and therapies. For example, a recent genome-wide association study of 2780 cases and 47,486 controls identified 12 genome-wide susceptibility loci which were significant for hypertrophic cardiomyopathy（HCM）（肥厚型心肌病）, and found that single-nucleotide polymorphism（多态性）heritability indicated a strong polygenic influence, especially for sarcomere-negative HCM（64% of cases; $h2g = 0.34 \pm 0.02$）. Another recent study of patients with hereditary transthyretin（TTR）（遗传性转甲状腺素）cardiac amyloidosis（心肌淀粉样变性）with polyneuropathy showed that administration of NTLA-2001 led to a decrease in serum TTR protein concentrations through targeted knockout of TTR. Hence, genetic screening of TTR may, thus, prove to be increasingly useful in the future as it may allow susceptible patients to be identified and treated appropriately at an earlier stage of disease. On the other hand, genetic testing in polygenic CVDs, with their

inherently more complicated genetic etiology(病因学), remains challenging.

2. Artificial intelligence（AI）is a discipline of computer science that aims to mimic human thought processes, learning capacity, and knowledge storage. A central tenet of AI is learning the value of potential choices rather than rigidly following predetermined thresholds(阈值) or procedures, e. g., optimizing the selection of variants to maximize the predictive accuracy for disease risk rather than using a predetermined list. AI involves several components, including machine learning and deep learning, with increasing potential to explore novel CVD genotypes(基因型) and phenotypes(显型), among many other exciting opportunities. In this review, we summarize several important current limitations of genomics(基因组学); provide a brief overview of AI; and identify the current applications, limitations, and potential future directions of AI in cardiovascular genetics.

3. The majority of CVDs and cardiovascular risk factors have a significant genetic component, which is most commonly polygenic in origin. Current clinical practice utilizes a patient's medical history, family history, physical examination, cardiac biomarkers, and various modalities of cardiac imaging to establish diagnoses and to stratify risks. Despite rapid advances and availability of genetic testing panels, clinicians seldom utilize genetic testing as part of their initial patient assessments beyond cases with a known family history of genetic, inherited CVDs (e.g., HCM, arrhythmogenic right ventricular cardiomyopathy（ARVC）(致心律失常性右心室心肌病), long QT syndrome（LQTS）(长QT综合征), or catecholaminergic polymorphic ventricular tachycardia（CPVT）(儿茶酚胺敏感性多形性室性心动过速)). This lack of routine testing as part of care pathway creates a "diagnostic gap" that can lead to inappropriate or ineffective treatment in patients suffering from inherited CVDs. In a recent study from Baylor College of Medicine's Human Genome Sequencing Center, 84% of surveyed physicians reported medical management changes, including specialist referrals, cardiac testing, and medication changes, after receiving the results of a panel of genes associated with CVDs.

4. Despite its demonstrated clinical relevance, current guidelines only recommend genomic testing for a small number of cardiac conditions, limited by the relatively few genetic tests that are currently available and the lack of strong studies in cardiovascular(心血管的) genetics. For example, Brugada syndrome has a large number of potentially pathogenic genetic variants but current guidelines continue to recommend a comprehensive genetic analysis for only Brugada syndrome caused by the SCN5A genetic variant. With advancements in genetic testing technologies, preemptive genetic testing for various cardiomyopathies may be useful in the presence of an asymptomatic(无临床症状的) type 1 Brugada ECG pattern, family history of dilated cardiomyopathy, or the development of spontaneous coronary artery dissection (SCAD)(自发性冠状动脉夹层). While a recent study by Murdock and colleagues

demonstrated the diagnostic potential of genetics guided coronary artery disease (CAD) risk factor management based on LPA polymorphisms and polygenic risk，genetic testing for a selection of well-understood variant-phenotype associations remains very limited（i. e., a "treatment gap"）. With further research and development，comprehensive genetic testing could become routinely used in clinical cardiovascular practice and applied to primary disease prevention and the facilitation of precision cardiovascular medicine.

5. Genomics is becoming nearly ubiquitous in biomedical research. Large-scale sequencing efforts have revolutionized our understanding of the complex genetic interrelationships involved in the pathogenesis（发病机制） of most cardiovascular conditions. The tremendous advancements in genomic research are largely driven by the advent of NGS，which has led to the discovery of novel associations and the ability to more easily assess genetic heterogeneity across patients. Several categories of NGS include：（1）whole genome sequencing（WGS）（全基因组测序）；（2）whole exome sequencing（WES）（全外显子组测序），where the sequencing is concentrated over the protein-coding regions of the genome（～2% of the genome）；and（3）gene panels，where very deep coverage（＞100× coverage）is generated for a select number of genes. Both WGS and WES allow for the accurate identification of single-nucleotide variants（SNVs）（单核苷酸变异），large copy number variations（CNVs）（拷贝数变异），small insertion deletions（InDels），and information on variant frequencies in different populations. Because WGS examines the noncoding regions of the genome，it offers a more comprehensive appraisal of both small and large genomic risk variants for CVDs. However，WGS is more costly and time consuming than WES，and may be limited by lower depth. Conversely，the results of WES，while more limited in scope，are typically viewed as more straightforward to interpret and historically have been a useful method to identify variants causing Mendelian disease. Panel-based NGS relies on high sequencing depth of previously determined important genetic loci，making this kind of testing more resource-efficient. However，the narrow focus of this type of assay results in decreased power to detect novel associations and is often less effective for assessing other types of genetic alterations，such as structural variants. Although NGS is now widely used due to its speed，robustness，and cost-effectiveness，orthogonal（正交的）confirmation with the traditional Sanger sequencing method is sometimes still required for validation prior to clinical use.

6. Nonetheless，the implementation of AI to NGS and genomics has already been shown to accurately predict the consequences of genetic risk factors in CVDs，show the noncoding-variant effects in CVDs，find patients with cardiac amyloidosis，and initiate specific therapies from tumor sequencing by integrating with electronic health records（EHRs）（电子健康记录）in several academic and medical institutions. Additionally，there are several direct-to-consumer genomics companies that use AI

along with WGS and WES; however, to date, these applications have been limited by a lack of transparency in the algorithms they utilize due to their proprietary nature and commercial competition, as well as a lack of a consistent validation cohort, genomic guided clinical trials, and high-quality phenotype data that are consistently encoded and managed. Although some direct-to-consumer companies have collaborated with academic institutions and published their methodologies, evidence for their clinical relevance remains scarce.

7. AI encompasses a broad range of applications for automated reasoning and inference, and is starting to have a major impact on clinical assessment and diagnosis. For example, in both United States of America (US) and United Kingdom (UK) datasets, AI outperformed human radiologists in screening mammography(乳房X线照相术) and significantly reduced false positives and false negatives. The most widely used groups of methods for pattern recognition in genomics include machine learning (ML) and deep learning (DL). Other AI approaches, for example natural language processing (NLP)(自然语言处理) and cognitive computing, are also starting to play a role in cardiovascular clinical care to enable more natural interactions between clinicians and computational systems.

From Life(*Basel*),*2022*,*12*(*2*)

After reading

Task 8   Build your vocabulary.

Directions: Match the following words with their corresponding definitions and Chinese equivalents.

English: cardiovascular   polymorphisms   cardiac   vessel   monogenic   polymorphism   sarcomere   catecholaminergic   cardiomyopathy

Chinese: 心血管的   遗传多态性   心脏的   （人或动物的）血管   单基因的   多型现象   肌原纤维节   儿茶酚胺能   心肌病

Paras. 1—7

English	Chinese	Definition
1. _____	_____	a. connected with the heart and the blood vessels (= the tubes that carry blood around the body)

2. _____　　_____ 　b. the occurrence of more than one form of individual in a single species within an interbreeding population

3. _____　　_____ 　c. connected with the heart or heart disease

4. _____　　_____ 　d. a tube that carries blood through the body of a person or an animal, or liquid through the parts of a plant

5. _____　　_____ 　e. of or relating to an inheritable character that is controlled by a single pair of genes

6. _____　　_____ 　f. the genetic variation within a population that natural selection can operate on

7. _____　　_____ 　g. one of the segments into which a myofibril is divided

8. _____　　_____ 　h. involving, liberating or mediated by catecholamine

9. _____　　_____ 　i. a disorder (usually of unknown origin) of the heart muscle (myocardium)

Guiding to learn

Task 9　Learn the following general academic vocabulary from the word bank.

assumption available distribute interpretation variable vary relevant restriction transfer criteria exclusion initial reliably validate adequate attribute emerging ethnicity compounded enforcement entity version capability incorporate transformation utilization coupled hierarchical intervention detection visualized coherence revolutionize

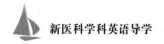

Beginning to read

Task 10   Now read the text.

Text C

Artificial Intelligence in the Diagnosis and Detection of Heart Failure: the Past, Present, and Future

Farah Yasmin et al

1. Artificial Intelligence（AI）possesses the capability to perform human intelligence-dependant tasks such as receiving perspicuity, learning semantics, and formulating an analysis using various algorithms and cognitive computing. AI uses the concept of Learning, which can be classified into supervised, unsupervised, and re-enforcement. Machine Learning（ML）is the core of AI that uses a model based on training data to make decisions, and program algorithms to solve the problem. The commonly utilized classification models include Binary, Multi-class, Multi-label and Imbalanced Classification. Binary classification uses algorithms like Logistic Regression（逻辑回归）, k-nearest neighbors, decisions tree, support vector machine and naïve bayes（朴素贝叶斯）to classify two labels' tasks. Multi-class uses algorithms like decisions tree, support vector machine, naïve bayes, random forest, and gradient boosting to classify tasks involving more than two labels. Multi-label classifies tasks that have two or more class labels, where one or more class labels may be predicted for each example, unlike the multi-class where a single class label is predicted for each example. The class labels with unequally distributed tasks are classified using the Imbalanced classification model. The distributions can vary from slightly imbalanced to severely imbalanced. It constitutes a significant challenge in predictive modelling as algorithms used for imbalanced classification are based on assumptions. Class labels are often string values, e.g., "spam", "not spam", which are mapped to numeric values in the process of label encoding. Deep Learning（DL）is a class of the ML algorithm that uses higher level features such as neural networks derived from a model of the human brain which allows a computer system to read, build, and learn complex hierarchical representation. It involves the transformation of the input data into a more compounded output data. Genetic predisposition（遗传倾向）is a major factor in the development of cardiovascular diseases such as atherosclerosis and advanced techniques such as the use of DL networks can be used to predict advanced coronary artery

calcium through a large-scale genome-wide association study. DL can be further subdivided into Artificial Neural Network，Convolutional Neural Network（卷积神经网络）, and Recurrent Deep Learning，as shown in Fig. 1. Table 1 illustrates the description of the functions of various components of artificial intelligence.

2. The evolution in cardiovascular diseases requires advancements in the treatment and diagnostic techniques，thus AI is now being rapidly incorporated in the field of cardiovascular medicine. AI has the potential to revolutionize the medical diagnosis，treatment，risk prediction，clinical care，and drug discovery through the interpretation of vast databases more efficiently as compared to the human brain. The use of DL-based diagnostic modalities such as cardiac angiography（心脏血管造影），echocardiography，and electrocardiogram （ECG）（心电图）in the field of cardiovascular medicine has played a pivotal role in revolutionizing the diagnosis of cardiovascular disorders such as heart failure，myocardial infarction，arrhythmia，and valvular heart disease. Paroxysmal Supraventricular Tachycardia（PSVT）（阵发性室上性心动过速）is a sporadic，sudden，and recurrent cardiovascular disorder that can worsen the quality of life of the patients. Although treatable；the condition is difficult to diagnose due to its instantaneous episodes occurring during normal sinus rhythm. However，the use of DML-based ECG has made the early diagnosis of PSVT possible. The use of diagnostic modalities and other AI-based tools such as medical resonance imaging（MRI），intravascular ultrasound，optical coherence tomography（OCT）（光学相干断层扫描），and single photon emission computed tomography（SPECT）（单光子发射计算体断层成像术）allows clinicians to make a detailed and faultless diagnosis of potentially fatal cardiovascular diseases. Furthermore，the use of ML-based AI has proven to predict 5-yearsurvivalrate in patients with cardiovascular diseases，more accurately（80%）as compared to the clinicians（60%）.

3. Heart failure（心力衰竭）is a major cardiovascular disorder with the mortality following hospitalization being 10.4% at 30 days，22% at 1 year，and 42.3% at 5 years，despite marked improvement in medical and device therapy. The multifactorial pathophysiology of HF that includes structural and functional abnormalities makes the diagnosis and treatment of HF more difficult. The advent of AI in the field of cardiovascular medicine through diagnostic modalities such as ECG，Echo，angiography，and the use of modern techniques like robotic percutaneous coronary intervention（机器人经皮冠状动脉介入治疗）in its management has markedly reduced the mortality of patients with HF. It is unlikely that AI will replace physicians，however，AI can act as an essential tool that can help physicians improve their clinical judgment，and provide a precise diagnosis of diseases like HF. In this study，we aim to discuss the role of AI in the detection and diagnosis of HF. We have also discussed the limitations in the incorporation of AI in cardiovascular medicine，and how it can be further developed.

From Reviews in Cardiovascular Medicine，2021，22（4）

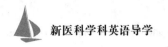

New words and expressions

subtype /ˈsʌbˌtaɪp/ *n.* a secondary or subordinate type or genre, esp a specific one considered as falling under a general classification 类型;次类型

mortality /mɔːˈtæləti/ *n.* the number of deaths in a particular situation or period of time 死亡数量;死亡率

electrocardiogram /ɪˌlektrəʊˈkɑːdiəʊɡræm/ *n.* If someone has an electrocardiogram, doctors use special equipment to measure the electric currents produced by that person's heart in order to see whether it is working normally. 心电图

hierarchical /ˌhaɪəˈrɑːkɪk(ə)l/ *adj.* arranged in a hierarchy 按等级划分的;等级制度的

transformation /ˌtrænsfəˈmeɪʃ(ə)n/ *n.* a complete change in sth (彻底的)变化,转变

predisposition /ˌpriːdɪspəˈzɪʃ(ə)n/ *n.* a condition that makes sb/sth likely to behave in a particular way or to suffer from a particular disease (易患某种病的)体质

atherosclerosis /ˌæθərəʊsklɪəˈrəʊsɪs/ *n.* a stage of arteriosclerosis involving fatty deposits (atheromas) inside the arterial walls, thus narrowing the arteries 动脉粥样硬化(症)

calcium /ˈkælsɪəm/ *n.* a chemical element. Calcium is a soft silver-white metal that is found in bones, teeth and chalk 钙

myocardial /ˌmaɪəʊˈkɑːdɪəl/ *adj.* of or relating to the myocardium 心肌的

arrhythmia /əˈrɪðmɪə/ *n.* an abnormal rate of muscle contractions in the heart 无节律性;心律不齐(失常)

sporadic /spəˈrædɪk/ *adj.* happening only occasionally or at intervals that are not regular 偶尔发生的;间或出现的;阵发性的;断断续续的

instantaneous /ˌɪnstənˈteɪnɪəs/ *adj.* happening immediately 立即的;立刻的;瞬间的

sinus /ˈsaɪnəs/ *n.* any of the hollow spaces in the bones of the head that are connected to the inside of the nose 窦;窦道

ultrasound /ˈʌltrəsaʊnd/ *n.* a medical process that produces an image of what is inside your body 超声波扫描检查

photon /ˈfəʊtɒn/ *n.* a unit of electromagnetic energy 光子;光量子

hospitalization /ˌhɒspɪtəlaɪˈzeɪʃn/ *n.* insurance that pays all or part of a patient's hospital expense (保证偿付住院费的)住院保证单

After reading

Task 11   **Build your vocabulary. Choose one word which can be used to replace the language shown in bold without changing the meaning of the sentence from the list below. Change forms and cases when necessary.**

ambiguity(*n.*)   annual(*adj.*)   construe(*v.*)   displace(*v.*)   efficient(*adj.*)
innate(*adj.*)   material(*n.*)   orbit(*v.*)   residue(*n.*)   reverberate(*v.*)   suspend(*v.*)

1. Data were maintained by the Department of Healthcare Quality Assessment, Tokyo University, Tokyo, Japan, which produces **yearly** site-specific reports to JCVSD participants for outcome analyses and quality improvement.

   _____

2. MUAC is a familiar concept to health providers in regions with high levels of malnutrition and is a more **proficient** alternative to determining weight for height z-scores.

   _____

3. Conflict of Interest Statement: The authors declare that the research was conducted in the absence of any commercial or financial relationships that could be **viewed** as a potential conflict of interest.

   _____

4. We will deal here exclusively with T cells, but many different cell types from both the adaptive and **intrinsic** arms of the immune system are motile within the ECM.

   _____

5. For each sample trial, the black or white cylinder was **halted** above the submerged platform.

   _____

6. Supplementary material Supplementary **substance** is available at British Journal of Anaesthesia online.

   _____

7. Radiographic evaluation frequently reveals a large, locally advanced malignancy invading into the **circles** or intracranially.

   _____

8. Questions remain as to how COVID-19 **rebound** after Paxlovid treatment differs between the BA.5 and BA.2.12.1 subvariants.

   _____

9. In addition, reduced movement of the base of tongue and pooling of **remainder** in the vallecula and pyriform sinuses promote aspiration after the swallow.

   _____

10. Anesthesiologists confirmed that the tidal volume measured by the anesthetic machine was 7 mL/kg because the tilt of the head could **supplant** the LMA.

    _____

Further reading

Goyal，H.，Sherazi，S. A. A.，Gupta，S.，et al.（2022）. Application of Artificial Intelligence in Diagnosis of Pancreatic Malignancies by Endoscopic Ultrasound：A Systemic Review. *Therapeutic Advances in Gastroenterology*. 15(4).

Haq，I. U.，Chhatwal. K.，Sanaka，K.，et al.（2022）. Artificial Intelligence in Cardiovascular Medicine：Current Insights and Future Prospects. *Vascular Health and Risk Management*. 18(6).

Krittanawong，C.，Johnson，K. W.，Choi，E.，et al.（2022）. Artificial Intelligence and Cardiovascular Genetics. *Life*（*Basel*）. 12(2).

Nam. D.，Chapiro，J.，Paradis，V.，et al.（2022）. Artificial Intelligence in Liver Diseases：Improving Diagnostics，Prognostics and Response Prediction. *JHEP Reports*. 4(4).

Yasmin，F.，Shah，S. M. I.，Naeem，A.，et al.（2021）. Artificial Intelligence in the Diagnosis and Detection of Heart Failure：the Past，Present，and Future. *Reviews in Cardiovascular Medicine*. 22(4).

Unit 10
Artificial Intelligence in Treatment （I）

Guiding to learn

The successful use of artificial intelligence （AI） for diagnostic meet purposes has prompted the application of AI-based cancer imaging analysis to address other, more complex, clinical needs. This unit will describe the evolution of and opportunities for AI in oncology imaging, focusing on hand-crafted radiomic approaches and deep learning-derived representations, with examples of their application for decision support. This unit also address the challenges faced on the path to clinical adoption, including data curation and annotation, interpretability, and regulatory and reimbursement issues.

Discuss the following questions with your partners.

1. What advantages do AI-enabled predictive or prognostic imaging biomarkers can offer?
2. What are the roles of AI and big data in cardio-oncology and imaging?
3. Do you know any AI models for the diagnosis of cancer? What are they?

Task 1   Learn the following general academic vocabulary.

availability derivation financial procedure specifically computational distinct evaluated exclusively framework negative validation attribute emergence ethnicity implementation implications statistically status exposure perspective accurately discriminate initiation extraction intervention sultimate unique predominant prospective compatible conversely minimally supplementary

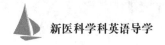

Beginning to read

Task 2　Now read the text.

Text A

Predicting Cancer Outcomes with Radiomics and Artificial Intelligence in Radiology

Kaustav Bera et al

1. In the past decade, drastic increases in computational power and memory have enabled the development and implementation of state-of-the-art artificial intelligence (AI) techniques for handling radiology images. We are currently witnessing increasing enthusiasm in this field, especially in oncology（肿瘤学） imaging, although computerized methods have been used in radiology since the 1960s. Early initiatives did not gain much traction because they relied on analogue image acquisition and limited computational resources. In the 1980s, the advent of digital imaging methods and improvements in computational architecture and storage renewed interest in these computer-aided detection (CAD)（计算机辅助检测） techniques. The initial success with AI in breast cancer detection paved the way for AI approaches to be used more broadly in diagnostic tasks such as tumour classification and cancer detection. Over the past decade, AI-based diagnostic tools have been continuously refined, and in many cases their diagnostic performance has been shown to match or even surpass that of human experts in multiple different cancer types. This success has led to AI approaches now being evaluated to aid more complex decision-making tasks, such as disease prognostication, prediction of response to different treatment modalities, recognition of treatment-related changes and discovery of imaging representations of phenotypic and genotypic features associated with prognosis.

2. In this Perspective, we exclusively focus on radiology AI-enabled biomarkers to predict disease outcome and response to treatment, with the ultimate goal of providing individualized management. We aim to equip clinicians interested in state-of-the-art AI approaches for decision-making in oncology with knowledge on the current novel tools being applied to outcome prediction, how these approaches are developed and, specifically, the types of image representation that can be used in AI applications. We discuss the clinical implications of AI in radiology（放射学） with regard to stratifying patients by disease severity and prognosis, predicting treatment response and benefit,

identifying unfavourable treatment outcomes from true disease progression，and non-invasively predicting salient molecular and genotypic（遗传型的）traits. First，we define AI-enabled imaging biomarkers and their use，contrasting them with existing biomarkers in oncology. We then focus on the general framework of AI-enabled imaging biomarkers，discussing the technical underpinnings of commonly used methods. We describe AI tools used in complex decision-making tasks，providing examples of how these AI indications have been used for the management of common cancer types. Finally，we conclude by summarizing some of the challenges and obstacles along the path towards clinical adoption of these approaches and by discussing future implications for oncology practice.

3. A biomarker is "a defined characteristic that is measured as an indicator of normal biological processes，pathogenic（致病的）processes or biological responses to an exposure or intervention，including therapeutic interventions". On the basis of the type of clinical decisions they can inform on，biomarkers can be grouped into several categories. In oncology，biomarkers have applications ranging from prevention，as is the case for biomarkers of cancer susceptibility or risk，to guiding high-level decision-making，among which prognostic and predictive biomarkers are the most clinically relevant.

4. A prognostic biomarker（预后生物标记）conveys information pertaining to the risk of a disease-related end point. In oncology，prognostic biomarkers are used to determine the risk profile of a patient with cancer on the basis of tumour characteristics. This knowledge enables the clinician to identify patients with poor prognosis who might be candidates for escalation of therapy and/or clinical trials. Conversely，if pre-emptively identified，patients with a good prognosis might have favourable outcomes with de-escalated therapy and could thus be spared the physiological and financial toxicities（毒性）of cancer treatment.

5. Most prognostic biomarkers currently used in oncology are molecular assays that rely on complex multigene signatures，such as Oncotype DX and MammaPrint in breast cancer（乳腺癌）and Decipher in prostate cancer（前列腺癌）. These genomic assays are included in the National Comprehensive Cancer Network（NCCN）（国家综合癌症网络）guidelines and are routinely used in clinical practice；however，they are prohibitively expensive and require tumour tissue obtained through an invasive procedure，thus limiting their availability and applicability in serial monitoring throughout treatment.

6. A predictive biomarker enables clinicians to make an informed management choice by identifying patients who would benefit from a particular therapeutic agent. In oncology，a biomarker is considered to be predictive if the treatment effect is statistically different in patients with biomarker-positive versus negative status. For example，in breast，gastric and gastro-oesophageal cancers（胃食管癌），among others，HER2 status serves as a biomarker for predicting the effectiveness of HER2-targeted

therapies，such as trastuzumab and pertuzumab. In non-small-cell lung cancer (NSCLC)(非小细胞肺癌)，the presence of EGFR(表皮生长因子受体) exon deletions or exon mutations serves as a biomarker of eligibility for treatment with EGFR tyrosine kinase inhibitors(酪氨酸激酶抑制剂)，such as osimertinib(奥西替尼) or erlotinib(厄洛替尼). Besides being prognostic, Oncotype DX is also a predictive biomarker validated in a prospective clinical trial to determine benefit from chemotherapy in women with early-stage breast cancer.

7. Rapid AI-driven advancements in computer vision and pattern recognition tasks have led to the emergence of AI-enabled imaging biomarkers. These biomarkers rely on the extraction of discriminating quantitative representations from radiology that capture properties of the tumour(肿瘤) phenotype that correlate with clinical outcomes. Two main categories of AI-enabled biomarker in radiology exist：hand-crafted radiomic and DL approaches. With hand-crafted radiomics，a set of representations are predefined by the AI development team that are composed of feature measurements with specific algorithmic derivations. These feature representations are then fed into a machine learning (ML) model，which in turn predicts an outcome. Some commonly used radiomic approaches focus on the various attributes of the area inside the tumour as well as the tumour microenvironment. Publicly available radiomics toolkits，enable researchers to apply hand-crafted radiomic features in their work without having to develop the feature pipeline themselves. In DL approaches，the development team defines a DL neural network that can be trained using a large data set to discover new representations that can be synthesized to predict a particular outcome.

8. AI-enabled predictive or prognostic imaging biomarkers can offer certain advantages over molecular assays. Given that they are assessed using routine clinical radiological scans(常规临床放射扫描)，AI-enabled imaging biomarkers are non-invasive, non-tissue-destructive, rapidly analysed, easily serialized, fairly inexpensive and fully compatible with existing clinical workflows，similar to AI-enabled pathology biomarkers，with the added advantage of being noninvasive. They additionally offer the ability to characterize a tumour over its full 3D volume，avoiding sampling errors that can occur with biopsy samples from heterogeneous tumours，as well as enabling the detection of changes in the TME(测温装置). Owing to these advantages over molecular testing, another category of AI-enabled biomarkers that reflect the genotype of a tumour has been developed using imaging representations，an approach known as radiogenomics(辐射基因组学). Radiogenomic approaches predictive of tumour mutational status could potentially become surrogate non-invasive biomarkers for established molecular biomarkers and could be applied in routine imaging. This approach would be similar to circulating tumour DNA-based liquid biopsy approaches，which are being developed as minimally invasive tools for cancer surveillance. Such

tests could also be used serially to detect changes in the predominant genotype of a tumour following initiation of treatment, a known cause of acquired resistance to targeted therapy that cannot be monitored accurately with invasive molecular testing.

From Nature Reviews Clinical Oncology，2022，19（2）

New words and expressions

decade /ˈdekeɪd/ *n*. a period of ten years 十年；十年期（尤指一个年代）

outcome /ˈaʊtkʌm/ *n*. the result or effect of an action or event 结果；效果

guideline /ˈɡaɪdlaɪn/ *n*. rules or instructions that are given by an official organization telling you how to do sth, especially sth difficult 指南；准则；指导方针；指导原则；行动纲领；参考

extraction /ɪkˈstrækʃn/ *n*. the act or process of removing or obtaining sth from sth else 提取；提炼；拔出

unique /juˈniːk/ *adj*. being the only one of its kind 唯一的；独一无二的；独特的；罕见的

minimally /ˈmɪnɪməli/ *adv*. something that is minimal is very small in quantity, value, or degree 最低限度地，最低程度地

predominant /prɪˈdɒmɪnənt/ *adj*. most obvious or noticeable 占优势的，主导的，支配的；普遍的，显著的；明显的；盛行的；最重要的，最强大的

prospective /prəˈspektɪv/ *adj*. expected to do sth or to become sth 预期的；潜在的；有望的；可能的；即将发生的；行将来临的

After reading

Task 3　Scan the text A again and answer the following questions.

1. What is biomarker?

2. What does a prognostic biomarker convey?

Task 4　Check your vocabulary. Fill in the blanks with the correct form of the words from the following box, each word can be used only once.

> anthropdogy（*n*.）　intimacy（*n*.）　foetus（*n*.）　province（*n*.）　render（*v*.）
> repress（*v*.）　quote（*v*.）　sift（*v*.）　triangle（*n*.）　surplus（*n*.）

1. In conducting this literature review I have learned, certainly, about the extent to which homosexuality has been researched in the fields of psychology, _____, history, and beyond.

2. Sanderson and Cantor (1995) examined the relationship between social dating goals

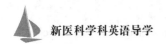

and effective sex education for individuals with different types of goals: establishing identity or establishing _____ .

3. Pregnant women who are heavy drinkers risk damaging the unborn _____ .

4. The Madras Presidency was a former _____ of the British Empire that included several districts in the southern region of India between latitudes 20° and 8°N and longitudes 74° and 86°E.

5. The employment of measures with populations for which measures were not intended can _____ research findings meaningless or misleading.

6. Although in zebrafish, Spg and Cas seem to cooperate in activation of sox17 expression, it is unclear if in mice early embryonic development, these two factors cooperate with each other in transcriptional activation of endoderm specific gene expression, or one may _____ the activity or expression of another.

7. A descriptive _____ of the process of developing Soul bonds is particularly illuminating for an argument I will make later.

8. Attempting to _____ through the literature on homosexuality, biology, and genetics can be daunting, so let us start simply.

9. When considering the epidemiologic _____ (agent, host, and environment), the best way to affect HIV transmission, with our current technology, is by breaking the chain between agent and host.

10. About the federal deficit Frank says, clearly we'd love to run a _____ instead of a deficit, but we're competing in a global market.

Task 5 Build your vocabulary. Read the sentences below, decide which word in each bracket is more suitable.

1. It remained very difficult to (procure/secure) food, fuel and other daily necessities.

2. An (Appendix/index) containing the skeletal report, with all chi-square calculations, can be found starting on the next page.

3. One part of her may feel the need to fit in and (assimilate/ingest) to the dominant culture while another part of her may feel committed to being a respected Navajo.

4. In contrast, misexpression of Hb in all neuro blasts resulted in extra MM-CB glia at the mid-line and a decrease in the number of mid-line (channel/deviate) glia.

5. It is hard to think that humans sprouted from trees but to incorporate this idea into a creationism (myth/legend) really speaks to how important the forest is to the entire Nordic culture.

6. Filling of any wetlands within the shore impact and secondary shoreline buffer zones shall be(embargoed/prohibited.)

7. To use my server, (append/affix) by the equation you want.

8. Current examinations of critical factors in CVD development often (diverge/

converge）on leptin.

9. Clinical research has demonstrated an association between（elevated/lifted）plasma leptin levels and cardiovascular complications in humans. One such study examined moderately hypercholesterolemic men with no history of myocardial infarction and/or coronary artery disease in an effort to identify new risk factors for CVD.

10. If the（angular/bent）velocity of a body changes，it is said to have an angular acceleration.

Guiding to learn

Task 6　Learn the following general academic vocabulary.

availability acquisition criteria reactive volume confer contrast overall parameter subsequently ratio accurate enhancement inhibit utility detection highlight intensity ongoing undergoing

Beginning to read

Task 7　Now read the text.

Text B

Multimodality Advanced Cardiovascular and Molecular Imaging for Early Detection and Monitoring of Cancer Therapy-Associated Cardiotoxicity and the Role of Artificial Intelligence and Big Data

Jennifer M Kwan et al

1. Cancer incidence is expected to increase by 50% by 2050, but over the past two decades, cancer mortality has improved in part due to earlier detection via screening and the advent of novel therapies such as tyrosine kinase inhibitors（TKI）（酪氨酸激酶抑制剂）for cancers like chronic myelogenous leukemia（CML）（慢性髓细胞白血病），liver, gastrointestinal and lung cancers, as well as immunotherapy, such as checkpoint inhibitors, for metastatic disease and an expanding list of indications including triple negative breast cancer, lung cancer, melanoma（黑素瘤），bladder cancer（膀胱癌），

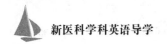

and renal cell cancer(肾细胞癌).

2. However，with the rise of newer oncologic therapies，there have been a spectrum of adverse cardiovascular toxicities including cardiomyopathy（CM）（心肌病），myocardial infarction(心肌梗死)，myocarditis(心肌炎)，arrhythmia(心律不齐)，hypertension（HTN）（高血压）and thrombosis(血栓症) that have been associated with these agents. More traditional cardiotoxic agents like anthracyclines(蒽环类药物)，one of the most widely used class of chemotherapeutics(化学疗法) due to improved overall cancer and survival outcomes has been shown to alter myocardial energetics，promote mitochondrial dysfunction(功能紊乱)，increase reactive oxygen species levels leading to activation of matrix metalloproteases(基质金属蛋白酶)，inhibit topoisomerase(拓扑异构酶) IIb and cause DNA strand breaks，thereby promoting cardiomyopathy .

3. HER2(人表皮生长因子受体2) inhibitors like trastuzumab(曲妥珠单抗) has also been shown to increase risk of CM via antagonizing important pro survival as well as other important signal transduction pathways for metabolism in the heart. Platinum agents like cisplatin(顺铂) have been shown to increase oxidative stress and increased apoptosis and has been associated with cardiomyopathy in rare instances. Alkylating（烷基化的）agents like cyclophosphamide（环磷酰胺），which can cause oxidative damage and direct endothelial cell damage have been linked to myocarditis and cardiomyopathy. Antimetabolites like 5 fluorouracil（5FU）（5氟尿嘧啶），which is commonly used in head and neck cancers as well as gastrointestinal cancers has been shown to increase risk of coronary vasospasm and myocardial infarction. Multiple myeloma therapies and vascular endothelial growth factor（VEGF）（血管内皮生长因子）inhibitors like bevacizumab(贝伐珠单抗) have been associated with thrombosis and hypertension by promoting endothelial cell dysfunction. TKIs(酪氨酸激酶抑制剂) like ibrutinib(依鲁替尼) has been associated with atrial fibrillation，while other TKIs such as ponatinib，sorafenib，sunitinib have been associated with CM and myocardial infarction（MI）.

4. Of the close to 2 million patients diagnosed with cancer in 2019，it is estimated that 38.5% are eligible for immune checkpoint inhibitors（ICI）（免疫检查点抑制剂）therapy. In addition to increased risk of myocarditis，pericarditis and vasculitis，ICI have been associated with increased risk of plaque rupture/acceleration of atherosclerosis(动脉粥样硬化) and thrombosis(血栓形成). ICI myocarditis is characterized by lymphocytic infiltration with CD4 and CD8 cells and mortality is high if not identified and if left untreated.

5. Newer immunotherapies may also increase risk of myocarditis，such as cellular therapies like CART(嵌合抗原受体T细胞免疫疗法) and molecular inhibitors such as CCR4(趋化因子受体) antagonist，mogamulizumab，which is used to treat T cell lymphomas. However，evaluation of the earliest signs of immune cell infiltration in the myocarditis process is limited. Imaging modalities like echocardiography（echo）and

magnetic resonance imaging（MRI）are routinely used to monitor and evaluate for the aforementioned oncologic therapy related cardiotoxicity，with both allowing for assessment of function and wall motion abnormalities and MRI allowing for additional tissue characterization using T1，T2，extracellular volume（ECV）（细胞外容积）and delayed gadolinium enhancement（DGE）（延迟钆增强）assessment. While nuclear studies like multi-gated acquisition（MUGA）scans have fallen out of favor for the evaluation of cardiomyopathy mediated by oncologic therapy due to the higher sensitivity，and availability of echo and MRI，emerging nuclear imaging using molecularly targeted radiotracers may confer more specificity and help elucidate the mechanisms of cardiotoxicity，many of which are already in clinical use for oncology purposes and thus can be adapted to evaluate their signal/role in cardiotoxicity. In addition to molecular targets，hyperpolarized MRI has emerged as a potential imaging modality to evaluate effects of oncologic therapy on cardiac metabolism and has reached human studies. Finally，artificial intelligence and big data of imaging modalities including electrocardiograms may be able to help predict and detect early signs of cardiotoxicity and response to cardioprotective（心脏保护）medications once cardiomyopathy develops but also help provide insights on diagnostic and prognostic value of molecular based imaging. We review current imaging modalities used to assess for cardiovascular toxicities associated with oncologic therapies and highlight ongoing research in the areas of molecular imaging，targeted molecular radiotracers and hyperpolarized MRI as well as the role of artificial intelligence（AI）and big data in imaging that would help improve detection，prognostication of oncologic therapy related cardiotoxicity.

6. Cardiotoxicity（心脏中毒）due to anthracycline use（often dose dependent，but can occur at any dose）are common，up to 5% with cumulative doses <400 mg/kg，but up to 20% for those treated with 700 mg/kg or more. HER2 inhibitor mediated cardiomyopathy can occur in 5%—10% of patients and is increased when given in conjunction with anthracyclines up to 27%. Oncologic therapy mediated cardiomyopathy can be evaluated by traditional imaging modalities such as echo and MRI，which are able to evaluate wall motion，left and right ventricular function and even early signs of toxicity via changes in strain，namely global longitudinal strain.

7. In addition to being the gold standard for volumetrics and ejection fraction，MRI has additional evaluation capabilities including tissue characterization for injured cells such as changes in ECV and increased native T1 times，shown with anthracycline use and increased T2 relaxation times with anthracycline toxicity. The presence of DGE post trastuzumab，a HER2 inhibitor，was associated with cardiomyopathy.

8. Feature tracking global longitudinal strain（GLS）（整体纵向应变）was first used in echo to show that it could be predictive of future cardiomyopathy in multiple studies of cancer patients undergoing cardiotoxic chemotherapy with anthracycline or

trastuzumab. For example，an increase in GLS ＞12 or 15% was associated with a significant drop in LVEF ＞ 10% 6 months after in several studies. MRI has subsequently shown that use of tagging，feature tracking strain or fast strain encoded （SENC） assessment are sensitive and highly accurate in detecting subclinical cardiotoxicity as evidenced by an increase in GLS for patients on cardiotoxic chemotherapy(化学疗法) such as anthracyclines，with SENC having a higher accuracy that was less dependent on loading conditions.

From Frontiers in Cardiovascular Medicine，2022，9（3）

After reading

Task 8   Build your vocabulary.

Directions：Match the following words with their corresponding definitions and Chinese equivalents.

English：promote   evaluation   acquisition   incidence   negative   subsequently   undergoing   visible   status   technique

Chinese：发生率   消极的   促进   评价   收购   随后   正在经历的   看得见的   地位   技巧

Paras. 1—7

English	Chinese	Definition
1. _____	_____	a. the extent to which sth happens or has an effect
2. _____	_____	b. bad or harmful
3. _____	_____	c. to help sth to happen or develop
4. _____	_____	d. act of ascertaining or fixing the value or worth of
5. _____	_____	e. the act of getting sth, especially knowledge，a skill，etc.
6. _____	_____	f. afterwards；later；after sth else has happened
7. _____	_____	g. to experience sth, especially a change or sth unpleasant
8. _____	_____	h. that can be seen
9. _____	_____	i. the legal position of a person, group or country
10. _____	_____	j. a particular way of doing sth

Guiding to learn

Task 9　Learn the following general academic vocabulary from the word bank.

> predominantly　scenario　simulating　revolutionary　accompany　accuracy
> intervention　reinforcement　qualitative　protocol　occurrence　manually
> concurrently　approximately　manipulation

Beginning to read

Task 10　Now read the text.

Text C

Artificial Intelligence in the Diagnosis and Management of Colorectal Cancer Liver Metastases

Gianluca Rompianesi et al

Colorectal cancer liver metastases

1. Colorectal cancer（CRC）（结肠直肠癌）is the most common gastrointestinal cancer，the third most frequently diagnosed malignancy（10.0%）overall，and the second highest cause of cancer-related deaths（9.4%），with incidences varying significantly worldwide. CRC development is predominantly sporadic，with patient age，environmental and genetic factors associated with a significantly increased risk. Over 20% of newly diagnosed CRC patients have distant metastases at presentation，with estimated 5-year survival dropping from 80%—90% in patients with local disease to a dismal 10%—15% in those with metastatic spread（转移扩散）. The liver is the preferential metastatic site，due to its anatomical proximity and the portal systemic circulation. This results in 25%—50% of CRC patients developing liver metastasis during the course of the disease. In cases of synchronous resectable colorectal cancer liver metastasis（CRLM）（结直肠癌肝转移），the treatment options range from the traditional staged approach，where the primary tumor is resected prior to systemic

chemotherapy and liver metastasis resection，to the combined approach of bowel and liver resection during the same procedure，or the "liver first" approach. Irrespective of the timing of the surgical resection，surgery in combination with chemotherapy is the optimal treatment for CRLM，but only 25% of patients are suitable candidates for resection at diagnosis. In patients not amenable to surgery，chemotherapy is the usual treatment of choice，with the potential to render 10%—30% of tumors technically resectable through a good response and downsizing. CRLM management is multidisciplinary，with oncologists，surgeons，radiologists and pathologists playing pivotal roles in the complex diagnostic and therapeutic decision-making processes aimed to achieve the best possible outcome for the patient. In such a complex oncological scenario(肿瘤场景)，with unsolved challenges in timely diagnosis，reliable prognostic factor identification and optimal treatment selection，there is a strong need for a precision-medicine，personalized approach in order to optimize patients' survival and quality of life. The recent progressive implementation of artificial intelligence （AI）in healthcare has been welcomed with enthusiasm by both healthcare professionals and the general public；however，there remain several issues which are yet to be solved. AI has the potential to overcome some of the current practice limitations，and to play a crucial role in all steps of the management of CRLM but its clinical benefits have yet to be clearly established and validated.

2. The aim of this review is to summarize and analyze the available evidence on the application of AI technologies in the diagnosis and management of patients affected by CRLM.

AI

3. The term AI encompasses all the possible applications of technologies in simulating and replicating human intelligence. These endless applications range from everyday life to finance and economics or various medical fields，thanks to the advances in computational power and the collection and storage of large amounts of data in healthcare. After being adequately programmed and trained，AI has the potential to outperform clinicians in some tasks in terms of accuracy，speed of execution and reduced biases. AI has therefore progressively demonstrated its potential across all human lifespan；from the optimization of embryo selection(胚胎优化选择) during in vitro fertilization(体外受精) to the prediction of all-cause mortality. The revolutionary potential of these technologies in healthcare has generated great interest in researchers，professionals and industries，with currently over 450 AI-based medical devices approved in Europe or the United States. Nevertheless，the surge of AI and its implementation in clinical practice has been accompanied by several issues including legal considerations regarding security and data，software transparency(软件透明度)，flawed algorithms and inherent bias in the input data.

Machine learning

4. The replication of human intelligence by AI with the utilization of data-driven algorithms（数据驱动算法）that have been instructed and self-train through experience and data analysis is generally defined as machine learning（ML）. After been programmed，ML can find recurrent patterns in large amount of appropriately engineered data and progressively learn and independently improve performance accuracy without human intervention. The ML algorithms are generally classified in supervised learning（监督学习）（the most frequent one，which utilizes classified data），unsupervised learning（where algorithms can independently identify patterns in data without previous classification），semi-supervised learning（半监督学习）（can use a combination of both labelled and unlabeled data）and reinforcement learning（强化学习）（uses estimated errors as proportional rewards or penalties to teach algorithms）. Deep learning（DL）is a class of ML techniques that has the ability to directly process raw data and perform detection or classification tasks automatically without the need for human intervention. The sets of algorithms utilized by DL are generally artificial neural networks（ANNs）constituted by several layers that elaborate inputs with weights，biases（or thresholds）and deliver an output. ML models can be combined with the large amount of qualitative and quantitative information mined from medical images（医学影像）（radiomics）and clinical data to assist clinicians in evidence-based decision making processes.

From World Journal of Gastroenterology，*2022*，*28*（*1*）

New words and expressions

security /sɪˈkjʊərəti/ *n*. the activities involved in protecting a country，building or person against attack，danger，etc. 安全；保护措施；安全工作

utilization /ˌjuːtəlaɪˈzeɪʃn/ *n*. the act of using 利用；应用；效用

intense /ɪnˈtens/ *adj*. very great；very strong 强烈的；激烈的；很大的

automatic /ˌɔːtəˈmætɪk/ *adj*. having controls that work without needing a person to operate them 自动的

acquisition /ˌækwɪˈzɪʃn/ *n*. the act of getting sth，especially knowledge，a skill，etc（知识、技能等的）获得，得到

enhancement /ɪnˈhɑːnsmənt/ *n*. the enhancement of something is the improvement of it in relation to its value，quality，or attractiveness 提高；增加；增强

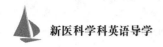

After reading

Task 11 **Build your vocabulary. Choose one word which can be used to replace the language shown in bold without changing the meaning of the sentence from the list below. Change forms and cases when necessary.**

inconsistent (*adj.*) ascribe (*v.*) assent (*n.*) comprise (*v.*) emanicipate (*v.*)
embrace (*v.*) enhance (*v.*) outcome (*n.*) saturate (*v.*) vague (*adj.*)

1. In all cases where the results were **at variance** with the hypothesis, alternatives hypotheses were proposed along with ideas for future investigation into the a posteriori hypothesis.   _____

2. There are always complicated interactions that determine decision-making and to **attributed** explanations from an outside perspective is extremely difficult.

    _____

3. Scholars now **cover** the idea that racism plays a key role in the differences in health care.

4. Slaves were not **liberate** until 1863 in the United States.   _____

5. If the desiccation response is necessary, then it is very possible to **boost** desiccation tolerance via genetic engineering or other biotechnological methods to increase production at low pressures.   _____

6. The latter institution, while certainly strong in ecological theory, does not, unlike the former, place such a strong emphasis on computer programming that its graduate school application largely **is composed of** an assessment of such skills.

    _____

7. The recruitment plan, consent and **agreement** processes and testing methods are described.   _____

8. Again, research to understand the mechanisms of bioinvasions could have helped predict this **result** and prevent implementation of such wasted efforts.

    _____

9. Decreasing soil moisture, particularly in **full to capacity** wet meadow tundra habitats, would increase decomposition rates and N-mineralization as soils become oxygenated.   _____

10. A nurse will often correctly predict that a patient has a specific problem based on a **uncertain** feeling, but when analyzed, that feeling is based on previous experience that is not simply the traditional cause and effect approach science usually relies on.

    _____

Further reading

Asiri, A. F., Altuwalah, A. S., et al. （2022）. The Role of Neural Artificial Intelligence for Diagnosis and Treatment Planning in Endodontics: A Qualitative Review. *The Saudi Dental Journal*. 34(4).

Bera, K., Braman, N., Gupta, A., et al. （2022）. Predicting Cancer Outcomes with Radiomics and Artificial Intelligence in Radiology. *Nature Reviews Clinical Oncology*. 19(2).

Kwan, J. M., Oikonomou, E. K., Henry, M. L., et al. （2022）. Multimodality Advanced Cardiovascular and Molecular Imaging for Early Detection and Monitoring of Cancer Therapy-Associated Cardiotoxicity and the Role of Artificial Intelligence and Big Data. *Frontiers in Cardiovascular Medicine*. 9(3).

Rompianesi, G., Pegoraro, F., Ceresa, C. D., e al. （2022）. Artificial Intelligence in the Diagnosis and Management of Colorectal Cancer Liver Metastases. *World Journal of Gastroenterology*. 28(1).

Zhao, W., Shen. L., Islam, M.T., et al. （2021）. Artificial Intelligence in Image-guided Radiotherapy: A Review of Treatment Target Localization. *Quantitative Imaging in Medicine and Surgery*. 11(12).

Unit 11
Artificial Intelligence in Treatment (Ⅱ)

Guiding to learn

In recent years, the popularity of artificial intelligence (AI) has made people's life more and more convenient. Artificial intelligence powered by the accumulating clinical and molecular data about cancer has fueled the expectation that a transformation in cancer treatments towards significant improvement of patient outcomes is at hand. This unit will introduce AI-driven diagnosis, AI-assisted identification, and AI-enabled improvement of cancer treatments.

Discuss the following questions with your partners.

1. What is machine learning?
2. What is artificial intelligence-driven diagnosis?
3. What is the AI-assisted identification?

Task 1　Learn the following general academic vocabulary.

available consistency complexity participatory regulatory constant criteria dominant framework illustrate insufficient proportion sequence sufficiently validation integration multidimensional regime fundamentally initiative intelligence utility dynamic inference successive eventual reinforcement terminal protocol intrinsic

Beginning to read

Task 2　Now read the text.

Text A

Can Artificial Intelligence Improve Cancer Treatments?
Youcef Derbal et al

1. The increasing burden of cancer on the capacity of healthcare systems and the need to reduce the negative impact of the disease and its treatment on the quality of life of cancer patients will require the development of cancer care strategies that are driven by predictive, personalized, preventive and participatory（P4）system approaches. Therein lies the catalysts towards achieving the necessary effectiveness and efficiency of cancer care delivery. Currently, the most widely used treatment strategies are informed by guidelines for clinical practice developed by expert panels. For example, through its Quality Oncology Practice Initiative, the American Society of Clinical Oncology（ASCO）(美国临床肿瘤学会) provides guidelines to oncology sites which in return report their practices. ASCO report back with an evaluation of the clinical site based on quality measures that focus on the process of care and patient-oriented measures such as pain management. However, with the increasing availability of big clinical and molecular data about cancer, artificial intelligence（AI）and machine learning（ML）are increasingly explored towards assisting in the multidimensional cancer treatment decision-making process. The potential utility of AI to oncology includes diagnostics, prognostications, treatment outcome predictions and treatment prescriptions. For instance, deep neural networks（DNNs）(深度神经网络) and convolutional neural networks have been used to classify skin cancer lesions and histologic patterns for lung cancer, predict HLA-peptide(人类白细胞抗原-肽) binding affinity for immunotherapy, and delineate target volume for radiotherapy. Other examples of ML applications in oncology include the assessment of short-term mortality risk of patients starting chemotherapy, breast cancer treatment recommendations to prevent metastasis, predictions of patients that can benefit from adjuvant therapy, and the use of Bayesian networks to assist in treatment decision-making. Predictions of cancer recurrence have also been made using Bayesian networks and logistic regression. Beyond these examples of AI application in oncology, AI may be indispensable to the future of precision oncology where the increasing number of

biomarkers and treatment options being available need to be considered in light of the continuously generated streams of clinical and molecular data to identify optimal treatments that would improve patient outcomes in the face of dynamic disease-treatment interactions. Furthermore，the effective realization of adaptive therapeutic modalities to counter cancer evolutionary dynamics and therapeutic resistance would benefit from AI-assisted therapy design approaches that mine big clinical and molecular data for actionable knowledge to assist in the synthesis of personalized，optimal cancer treatment regimes（最佳癌症治疗方案）.

2. The path to the realization of the AI potential in oncology is aligned with the drive for greater standardization，efficiency and consistency of cancer care across the various domains of the oncology（肿瘤学）workflow. This drive is best illustrated by the ongoing efforts invested towards the adoption of digital pathology and the use of AI in radiation oncology. However，there are significant challenges to the adoption of AI in the oncology clinic. These challenges range from the lack of data standardization and the insufficient availability of annotated data to the opacity of AI algorithms（人工智能算法）and their eventual performance drift due to the expanding cancer knowledge and data universe. Furthermore，the dearth of clinical validations（缺乏临床验证）of AI algorithms and the lack of adequate frameworks for regulatory and legal governance of patient data and AI algorithms are also notable barriers to the wide adoption of AI models in clinical decision-making. The development of standards，guidelines and frameworks for the clinical validation of AI are among the ongoing efforts to overcome the barriers to the integration of AI in clinical practice. For oncology，where a tangible impact of AI use on patient outcomes is proving to be difficult to achieve，more research is needed to study the extent to which AI supported treatment decision-making can improve cancer treatment.

3. ML algorithms are fundamentally built on data-driven machine learned mappings that represent correlations or causality between variables of interest. Learned or discovered correlations and patterns from big data are the basis for inferences，predictions，prescriptions and recommendations made by AI/ML algorithms. For non-safety critical applications such as image recognition，movie recommendations，market segmentation or trivia games，the use of AI has been very effective in mobilizing the statistical power of big data towards solving the problems at hand. On the other hand，replicating the success of AI to treatment decision-making in oncology has so far been elusive. Machine learned or discovered statistical correlations between treatments and patient outcomes are inevitably limited in their predictive power due to the reliance on temporal snapshots of tumor dynamics associated with treatment response data of the relevant patient population. Indeed，the heterogeneity（异质性）and evolutionary dynamics of cancer can potentially make every newly

diagnosed cancer sufficiently different from the machine learned statistical patterns for the AI algorithms to yield reliable inferences about treatment recommendations that can improve patient outcomes. In particular，the static data context of machine learning imposes an intrinsic limitation on the capacity of ML models to recapitulate the nonlinear，time-varying dynamics of patient treatment response. Furthermore，the longitudinal nature of cancer care requires AI algorithms to be adaptive to the inevitable changes of the tumor pathophysiology which occur during the multiple cycles of treatments administered in the neoadjuvant（新辅助疗法），curative，adjuvant，management and relapse settings. In light of cancer unique challenges that are highlighted above，further research is needed to chart feasible pathways towards realizing AI potential utility to cancer treatment decision-making.

4. The expanding universe of therapeutic options and the availability of growing clinical and molecular datasets about cancer are prime ingredients for realizing the vision of an AI-supported personalized，precision oncology. The potential utility of AI may be leveraged towards the development of an adaptive cancer treatment framework that addresses cancer evolutionary dynamics（癌症进化动力学），which underlies therapeutic resistance as the most critical challenge in the fight against cancer. The conception of such framework is inspired by the vision of rapid learning health care systems，where routinely collected and analyzed patient clinical and omics data can provide a constant source of updated clinical evidence to support the continuous improvement of treatments and patient health outcomes. Adaptive cancer treatment approaches require the integration of three canonical components of effective clinical decision-making：

- Modeling disease state dynamics(疾病状态动力学建模)
- Prediction of treatment outcomes and toxicity(毒性)
- Adaptive treatment recommendations

5. The consideration of the above-mentioned elements addresses key challenges associated with the complexity of decision-making in oncology. The structure of this nominal，clinical decision-making framework supports the inclusion of decision factors and criteria associated with the physician，the patient and the context of the oncology practice which are usually considered in making clinical decisions. These decision factors include patient disease features，biomarkers，treatment toxicity，treatment outcomes，patient quality of life，treatment protocols and guidelines，and physician experience. The consideration of tumor evolutionary dynamics through the modeling of disease state stems for the growing understanding of the determinant role that evolution has in the progression of cancer and the necessity to operationalize such insight to steer cancer dynamics away from therapeutic resistance（治疗耐药）. The regular monitoring and prediction of tumor evolutionary dynamics would enable the

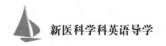

synthesis of adaptive treatment recommendations that are personalized to the specific features of the patient's disease and its progression dynamics.

From Health Informatics Journal, 2022, 28(2)

New words and expressions

participatory /pɑːˈtɪsɪpeɪtəri/ *adj*. affording the opportunity for individual participation 参与的；参与性的

catalyst /ˈkætəlɪst/ *n*. a substance that initiates or accelerates a chemical reaction without itself being affected 催化剂

oncology /ɒŋˈkɒlədʒi/ *n*. the branch of medicine concerned with the study and treatment of tumors 肿瘤学

multidimensional /mʌltɪdɪˈmenʃənl/ *adj*. having or involving or marked by several dimensions or aspects 多面的，多维的

prognostication /prɒgˌnɒstɪˈkeɪʃn/ *n*. a sign of something about to happen 预兆

histologic /hɪsˈtɒlədʒɪk/ *adj*. of or relating to histology 组织学的

affinity /əˈfɪnəti/ *n*. state of relationship between organisms or groups of organisms resulting in resemblance in structure or structural parts 亲和力；匹配度

delineate /dɪˈlɪnɪeɪt/ *vt*. show the form or outline of 描绘

opacity /əʊˈpæsɪti/ *n*. the quality of being opaque to a degree 不透明

validation /væliˈdeɪʃn/ *n*. finding or testing the truth of something 确认

tangible /ˈtændʒəbl/ *adj*. capable of being treated as fact 明确的；可感知的

elusive /ɪˈluːsɪv/ *adj*. be difficult to detect or grasp by the mind 难以捉摸的

determinant /dɪˈtɜːmɪnənt/ *n*. a determining or causal element or factor 决定子；决定因素

vulnerability /vʌlnərəˈbɪlɪti/ *n*. susceptibility to injury or attack 易损性

perturbation /ˌpɜːtəˈbeɪʃn/ *n*. a secondary influence on a system that causes it to deviate slightly 紊乱

After reading

Task 3   Read Text A again and answer the following questions.

1. What are challenges to the adoption of AI in the oncology clinic?
2. How much do you know about therapeutic resistance?

Task 4   Check your vocabulary. Fill in the blanks with the correct form of the words from the following box, each word can be used only once.

challenge（n.）   diameter（n.）   enable（v.）   expert（n.）   export（n.） fundamental（adj.）   import（n.）   luxury（n.）   pest（n.）   pollution（n.）   starve（v.） temporary（adj.）   tractor（n.）

1. The industry feels they are being undervalued and the consequence of increased ethanol production will result in loss to the economy because of their need to _____ agriculture byproduct.

2. Various ecological conditions have been claimed to _____ optimal evolution responsible for the recent spread of multiple subtypes and strains in multiple hosts.

3. One reason stems from the increased use of mechanized technology, which replaces poor laborers who work for little, with _____ and other machinery.

4. Developing new systems for different regions could be a major _____ to the widespread adoption of LIHD, requiring knowledge and expertise of local ecosystems and a great deal of research.

5. Therefore, the flea feels _____ and avidly seeks another blood meal from a new host.

6. He argues that the role of the government should be to support high value _____ and jobs, and promote industries within the U.S.

7. Monocultures of switchgrass or other grasses provide few niches for natural predators that feed on crop _____ , so chemical pesticides are often applied.

8. The weakness of this activity is the possibility that the activity level will return to its baseline after the competition is over, making this a _____ solution.

9. Cheyne believed that the modern world, with its imported _____ goods and city living, posed a great threat to the upper-class body, his included.

10. Streams in watersheds dominated by outwash will have a larger median particle size than streams in watersheds dominated by lacustrine because sand is larger in _____ than clay.

Task 5   Build your vocabulary. Read the sentences below, decide which word in each bracket is more suitable.

1. A similar effect can be observed in environmental systems: we are in danger of losing our global biodiversity to a monotonous（fate/destiny）.

2. During their hibernation, these hosts produced large amounts of glycerine, which was then overcome by the development of a glycerine fermentation（process/ action）in the plague bacterium.

3. This particular plant is especially conducive to scientific experiments involving photosynthesis because of its ability to produce oxygen（bubbles/blobs）as it carries

out photosynthesis, making it simple to monitor the rate of photosynthesis in an experiment.

4. Simon is instructed to develop attitudes and expectations towards Dr. G whether they are negative, (hostile/unfriendly), or positive.

5. I will begin with a discussion of the costs of benefits of dispersal, followed by a (catalogue/brochure) of the proximate causes of dispersal and their corresponding ultimate selective pressures.

6. Though such a policy program will likely face hard implementation problems across the spectrum, sufficient mandates and funding should (compel/urge) DOE to implement efficiently.

7. However, the danger of (theft/burglary) could also come from one's fellow travelers: he advises that pilgrims should get a padlock for the door of their chamber in the ship to protect their food and other provisions.

8. They experienced everything that they were hoping, but the constant anxiety of the trip becoming a bust has essentially (drained/emptied) much of the joy of the true experience.

9. Antibody-binding (sites/spots) of some subtypes of HA and NA have been described by X-ray crystallography and electron micrographs of monoclonal antibody escape mutants.

10. For example, younger individuals may be (inferior/worse) competitors and therefore more likely to emigrate to a new, lower-density patch.

Guiding to learn

Task 6　Learn the following general academic vocabulary.

consistency abnormal consumption distinction evaluation reconstruction conventional validate emergence integrate parameter exposure facilitate underlying dynamic extraction hierarchical intervention paradigm dramatic predominantly reinforcement manually trigger

Beginning to read

Task 7　Now read the text.

Text B

Artificial Intelligence-Driven Diagnosis of Pancreatic Cancer
Bahrudeen Shahul Hameed and Uma Maheswari Krishnan

1. Pancreatic cancer（PC）（胰腺癌）is among the most fatal and invasive tumors of the digestive system. It has been referred to as the "king of cancer", due to its aggressiveness, invasiveness and rapid metastasis, poor survival, and poor prognosis. Recent decades have witnessed a surge in the incidence of pancreatic cancer across the globe that has been largely linked to ageing, alcohol consumption, smoking, sedentary lifestyle, obesity, chronic pancreatitis, diabetes, hereditary factors, long-term exposure to air and water pollutants, unhealthy lifestyle, and diet. Surgery has been the main therapeutic intervention for these patients. However, several factors, including the absence of specific clinical manifestations and molecular markers, have resulted in the detection of the disease only at advanced stages, thereby making surgical options ineffective. Therefore, an early diagnosis and accurate stratification of pancreatic cancer stages are important for improved therapeutic outcomes. Pancreatic cancer diagnosis（胰腺癌诊断）is challenging because the pancreas is a deep-seated retro-peritoneal organ with complex surrounding structures. The highly vascularized environment surrounding the pancreas facilitates rapid metastasis of the cancer that makes pancreatic cancer highly aggressive. The common symptoms of pancreatic cancer include abdominal pain, changes in the consistency of faeces（粪便）, nausea（恶心呕吐）, bloated body, co-morbidities（共病）, such as diabetes and jaundice（黄疸）, abnormal liver function parameters, loss of weight, etc. These symptoms usually become prominent only during the advanced stage of the disease and are often missed during the early stages. Further, serological markers for pancreatic cancer, such as CA – 19 – 9, are not highly specific and indicate only the advanced stage of the disease, thereby increasing the mortality risk of the affected individual. Several imaging tools, including magnetic resonance imaging（MRI）, computed tomography（CT）, endoscopic ultrasound（EUS）（超声内镜）, etc., have also been explored for the diagnosis of pancreatic cancer. Due to rapid advances in recent years, imaging technology has emerged in the forefront for the diagnosis, staging, and prognosis of

pancreatic cancer. However，distinction of a cancerous lesion from other pancreatic disorders，such as pancreatitis，a chronic inflammation of the pancreas，remains a major roadblock in the accurate and early diagnosis of pancreatic cancer. Despite the existence of advanced imaging equipment，confirmation of pancreatic cancer is confirmed through biopsy after imaging. Not only is this time-consuming，but it also increases the probability of mortality in the affected individual，due to the inordinate delay. A study had reported that nearly 90% of the misdiagnosis of pancreatic cancer was due to the inability to identify the vascular invasion(血管侵犯) and the difficulty in spotting the underlying tumour mass，due to the inflammation.

2. Several approaches to improve the sensitivity and prediction accuracy of these imaging techniques have been reported in the literature. These include the use of image contrast agents to improve the resolution and sensitivity and the use of image processing software for a better diagnostic accuracy(诊断准确性). In recent years，the emergence of artificial intelligence and deep learning has transformed the landscape of an image-driven diagnosis of pancreatic cancer(胰腺癌的影像诊断)with a dramatic improvement in the prediction accuracy. The various attempts to integrate artificial intelligence for the diagnosis of pancreatic cancer are discussed in the following sections.

3. The advances in computer technology，witnessed in the recent decades，coupled with the development of effective image processing strategies，have ushered in a new era of "digital medicine". As a result，clinical personnel can avoid the laborious medical image analysis performed manually，thus saving time as well as overcome errors in diagnosis arising，due to the differences in expertise and clinical exposure. The 21st century has witnessed the widespread use of artificial intelligence (AI)(人工智能) that employs computer programs to perform tasks associated with human intelligence，such as learning and problem-solving. The phrase "artificial intelligence" was first coined by John McCarthy in the mid-1950s，and has since evolved from a set of 'if-then' commands to more complex algorithms(复杂算法) that mimic the human brain in some aspects. The application of AI tools has resulted in the emergence of a new field of clinical diagnosis，namely，precision oncology that uses a large volume of data from genomics，proteomics，and metabolomics. AI-based cancer diagnosis is mainly driven by machine learning (ML) and deep learning (DL) techniques. Machine learning uses computational methods to analyse large volumes of data and identify patterns for prediction. ML can be supervised where it uses data from previous trials/measurements for the identification of patterns or trends for making predictions.

4. Another type of ML that is yet to be applied for cancer diagnosis，is reinforcement learning where the algorithm uses the data to understand and respond to the environment predominantly by a trial-and-error process(试错过程). In other words，reinforcement learning is an advanced concept that could also facilitate

decision-making, in addition to prediction. Thus, apart from a diagnosis of pancreatic cancer, reinforcement learning could be used to alert clinicians（临床医生）in remote locations or trigger actuators for releasing a therapeutic agent. These concepts, though attractive, are yet to be realized, but could very well represent the diagnostic technology of the future. Deep learning is another sub-type of AI that uses large data sets and complex algorithms that mimic the human brain to enable prediction, forecasting, and decision-making. Most of the DL is supervised and uses data for training for the decision-making process, unlike reinforcement learning that is a dynamic process which relies on a trial-and-error method for the same. Both DL and reinforcement learning（强化学习）are advanced concepts that require a longer duration for training and testing.

5. A plethora（多血症）of supervised and unsupervised ML and DL models continue to be developed and explored for improving the accuracy of a pancreatic cancer diagnosis at the early stage which could be invaluable in enhancing the survival of the affected individual. The complexity of the algorithms will reflect the type of functions they can perform ranging from feature extraction, simple clustering or segregation of data, classification of data, prediction, forecasting, and decision-making. Algorithms such as Naïve-Bayes（朴素贝叶斯）, support vector machine, linear regression analysis, ensemble methods, decision tree, K-mode, hidden Markov model, hierarchical, Gaussian mixture, and neural networks have all been explored with different imaging data sets for distinguishing cancerous tissue from non-cancerous tissues.

6. The classification of images for diagnosis using various AI models can be broadly divided into one-stage and two-stage methods. The one-stage method segments the medical image into grids and applies the model for classification while the two-stage method demarcates several candidate zones that are used for classification during the training. Though time-consuming, the two-stage object method identifies and screens regions of interest resulting in more accurate predictions. Region-based convolution network（R-CNN）（区域卷积网络）, Fast R-CNN, and Faster R-CNN have been employed in the two-stage method as an integrated network for discriminative feature extraction, segmentation, and classification for an improved cancer detection without compromising the spatial structures.

7. Medical imaging has been widely used for locating and diagnosing cancerous tissue in the gastrointestinal tract（胃肠道）. Current analysis is largely dependent upon the expertise and experience of the clinician. The quality of the images also influences the diagnosis through conventional methods. The field of digital pathology continues to evolve from the first generation of image processing that involved the use of image processing tools to analyse a single slide, to much more advanced second-generation tools that could scan, analyse, and store records of whole tissue samples. The current

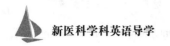

paradigm in digital pathology（病理学）involves the use of AI-based algorithms to analyse images，diagnose the condition with a high accuracy，and even predict the possibility of developing the disease even before the onset of the disease.

From Cancers（Basel），2022，14（21）

After reading

Task 8   Build your vocabulary.

Directions：Match the following words with their corresponding definitions and Chinese equivalents.

English：manifestation   prominent   mortality paradigm usher   reinforcement   supervise   segregation   spatial   extraction   hierarchical

Chinese：显著的   引导   表现   分离   范式   必死性   分层级的   监督   空间的   增强   提取

	English	Chinese	Definition
1.	_____	_____	a. keep an eye on
2.	_____	_____	b. the quality or state of being mortal
3.	_____	_____	c. a device designed to provide additional strength
4.	_____	_____	d. having a quality that thrusts itself into attention
5.	_____	_____	e. relating to space and the position，size, shape, etc. of things in it
6.	_____	_____	f. an appearance in bodily form
7.	_____	_____	g. the act of separating people or things from a larger group
8.	_____	_____	h. show（someone）to their seats，as in theaters or auditoriums
9.	_____	_____	i. a typical example or pattern of sth
10.	_____	_____	j. arranged in a hierarchy
11.	_____	_____	k. the act or process of removing or obtaining sth from sth else

Guiding to learn

Task 9   Learn the following general academic vocabularies from the word bank.

> approximately variant prospective identification accumulation consequent
> inhibit available retain consequent complement evolution proportion
> capable consistent

Beginning to read

Task 10   Now read the text.

 Text C

The AI-Assisted Identification and Clinical Efficacy of Baricitinib in the Treatment of COVID－19

Peter J. Richardson et al

1. The COVID－19 pandemic has caused the death of approximately 6 million people, with a case fatality rate which may be as high as 20% in those over 80 years old. Vaccines have proved to be extremely effective in reducing the damage and hospitalisation caused by this infection, although some patients still need supportive care. As the SARS-CoV－2 virus has continued to evolve, the potential for the virus to escape vaccine and exposure induced immunity remains a threat. In this situation, as at the start of the pandemic when no such vaccines were available, it is important that there exist therapeutics for the treatment of severely ill patients. This review described the identification, mechanism of action, and validation of the already approved rheumatology drug（风湿病药物）baricitinib as a treatment for hospitalised patients with COVID－19. In addition, comparison with other agents demonstrates that this drug is the most potent of the immune modulators（免疫调节）in reducing COVID－19 mortality. As a result, it is now strongly recommended for the treatment of COVID－19 by the WHO.

2. Infection by SARS-CoV－2 is usually via respiratory droplets（通过呼吸道飞沫）

and，like the related SARSCoV－1 and MERS viruses，results in a biphasic disease. The first phase shows mild symptoms，e.g.，fever，muscle pains，fatigue，headache，diarrhoea，loss of taste and smell，and a cough which may last for up to 2 weeks. This is the experience of most patients，but in some this phase is followed by the onset of breathlessness and pneumonia，often requiring oxygen therapy，and which can also be associated with severe pulmonary and systemic inflammation，similar to a cytokine storm（细胞因子风暴）. This involves high levels of circulating cytokines with widespread organ damage，vascular damage/thrombosis，and acute respiratory distress syndrome（ARDS）（急性呼吸窘迫综合征）. It is unclear why some people suffer from this hyper-inflammatory episode while others do not. Perhaps the most common explanation is that in those experiencing severe disease the response of both the innate and adaptive immune systems is dysregulated. This dysregulated response is associated with ageing of the immune system，obesity，and with chronic underlying diseases such as cardiovascular disease，diabetes，COPD，and others.

3. The pathophysiological mechanisms（病理生理机制）implicated in COVID－19 include virus induced cytopathy，hypertension from virus induced internalisation of its receptor ACE2，hyper-inflammation including cytokine and complement activation，cell death from excessive cytokines（pyroptosis），hypercoagulation（高凝状态），and perhaps autoimmunity. The endothelial lining of the microvasculature appears particularly hard hit，probably due to a combination of factors including ACE2 expression with consequent virus infection，microthrombosis，and innate immune activation（先天免疫激活） with neutrophil and macrophage activation and extravasation.

4. Ageing，the major risk factor for severe COVID－19，results in the accumulation of a number of defects in the innate and adaptive immune systems. For example，the number of T and B lymphocytes，macrophages，granulocytes，and lymphatic follicles（淋巴滤泡） are significantly creased in the elderly. Ageing macrophages and granulocytes（衰老的巨噬细胞和粒细胞） adopt an enhanced inflammatory state secreting pro-inflammatory cytokines，and showing impaired phagocytosis，migration，and clearance，thereby compromising the ability of these cells to clear infections and damage. Thus，the aged cells of the innate immune system generate a proinflammatory state（so called "inflammaging"）associated with reduced clearance of virus and virus-infected cells. This may also be associated with the accumulation of senescent cells in other tissues where they secrete a range of mediators known as the senescence-associated secretory phenotype（or SASP）（衰老相关分泌表型）. These mediators include many proinflammatory cytokines which may also contribute to inflammaging.

5. Despite the low-grade inflammation seen in the aged，the development of excessive numbers of terminally differentiated T cells，with a paucity of naïve T cells

has been observed（a condition known as immunosenescence）（免疫衰老）. The relative lack of naïve T cells compromises the ability of the aged immune system to mount a defence against novel pathogens such as SARS-CoV‑2. Increased numbers of senescent T cells are also associated with autoimmune disease（自身免疫疾病），chronic viral infection，as well as the reduced response to vaccines seen in the aged. These cells show increased NK receptor，granzyme B，and perforin expression and have lost antigen-specific cell killing but retain a strong nonspecific killing potential.

6. Intriguingly，senescent T cells are also associated with some of the underlying medical conditions which increase the risk of severe COVID‑19 disease. In rodent models（啮齿模型），senescent T cells can induce diabetes and obesity，while their clearance moderates the disease. It is therefore tempting to speculate that one reason for the susceptibility of the aged，and those with chronic diseases such as rheumatoid arthritis and diabetes，is due to the higher prevalence of senescent cells（衰老细胞）in these patients，including those of the immune system. Similarly，T cell immunosenescence is closely related to the development of cardiovascular disease，another chronic disease state associated with susceptibility to severe COVID‑19 disease. However the role，if any，of senescent T cells in the susceptibility of the aged to SARS-CoV‑2 has yet to be proven.

From Vaccines（Basel），2022，10（6）

New words and expressions

biphasic /baɪˈfeɪzɪk/ *adj*. having two distinct phases 二相的，双相性的

symptom /ˈsɪmptəm/ *n*. any sensation or change in bodily function that is experienced by a patient and is associated with a particular disease 症状

diarrhoea /daɪəˈrɪə/ *n*. a symptom of infection or food poisoning or colitis or a gastrointestinal tumor 腹泻

vascular /ˈvæskjʊlə(r)/ *adj*. of or relating to or having vessels that conduct and circulate fluids 血管的

innate /ɪˈneɪt/ *adj*. present at birth but not necessarily hereditary 天生的；先天的

internalisation /ɪnˌtɜːnəlaɪˈzeɪʃən/ *n*. learning（of values or attitudes etc.）that is incorporated within yourself 内化

extravasation /ɪkˌstrævəˈseɪʃən/ *n*. the process of exuding or passing out of a vessel into surrounding tissues 外渗物；溢出

senescent /sɪˈnesnt/ *adj*. growing old 衰老的

mediator /ˈmiːdieɪtə(r)/ *n*. a substance or structure that mediates a specific response in a bodily tissue 介质

susceptibility /səˌseptəˈbɪləti/ *n*. the state of being very likely to be influenced, harmed or affected by sth 易受影响的

antiviral /æntiːˈvaɪərəl/ *adj.* inhibiting or stopping the growth and reproduction of viruses 抗病毒的

pathogenic /pæθəˈdʒenɪk/ *adj.* able to cause disease 致病的

reproducible /riːprəˈdjuːsəb(l)/ *adj.* capable of being reproduced 可再生的

randomised /ˈrændəmaɪzd/ *adj.* set up or distributed in a deliberately random way 随机的；随机化的

After reading

Task 11　**Build your vocabulary. Choose one word which can be used to replace the language shown in bold without changing the meaning of the sentence from the list below. Change forms and cases when necessary.**

bulk (*n*.)	fluid (*n*.)	fulfil (*v*.)	huge (*adj*.)	inspect (*v*.)	instance (*n*.)
novel(*n*.)	revolve(*v*.)	shrink(*v*.)	switch(*v*.)	topic(*n*.)	vital(*adj*.)

1. As of now, it appears that cultural traits can, in this **case**, serve as the initial step towards speciation. _____

2. Tumor identification is possible because of differences in relaxation rates of **majority** water of normal tissues and tumors. _____

3. Weight loss is often dramatic during the first two to three weeks; this is because of the decreasing blood volume and **liquid** retention that has accumulated during pregnancy. _____

4. There has been virtually no coverage of the **subject** in major scientific journals, including those in parasitology. _____

5. After visually **examining** the pitch contours of the first-syllable-stressed token and the second-syllable-stressed token, the following design was chosen to modify the pitch contours. _____

6. If this sector slowly **changes** over to renewable energy, the impact on the renewable energy market would be tremendous, forcing more and more companies to invest in these new technologies allowing them to grow to heights that we could have only dreamed about a decade ago. _____

7. Reality is composed of a rather tenuous fabric in the catalogue of fantasy **stories** we have explored this semester. _____

8. It is almost a chore necessary to making babies and letting women **keep** their biologically defined destiny, rather than also being a pleasurable part of life and romantic relationships. _____

9. The dispute **rotates** around how land is used and how much influence local officials should have in managing those lands. _____

10. The isolation of virgin females and the ability to produce viable crosses with the selected flies was a **essential** piece in the overall goal of establishing a chromosomal map of unknown mutations. _____

Further reading

Bravo, J., Wali, A. R., Hirshman, B. R., et al. (2022). Robotics and Artificial Intelligence in Endovascular Neurosurgery. *Cureus*. 14(3).

Derbal, Y. (2022). Can Artificial Intelligence Improve Cancer Treatments? *Health Informatics Journal*. 28(2).

Hameed, B. S., Krishnan, U. M. (2022). Artificial Intelligence-Driven Diagnosis of Pancreatic Cancer. *Cancers (Basel)*. 14(21).

Richardson, P. J., Robinson, B. W. S., Smith, D. P., et al. (2022). The AI-Assisted Identification and Clinical Efficacy of Baricitinib in the Treatment of COVID-19. *Vaccines (Basel)*. 10(6).

Unit 12
Artificial Intelligence in Nursing

Guiding to learn

During the last decade, artificial intelligence has been widely applied to many fields. Research on technologies based on artificial intelligence in nursing has also increased, with applications showing great potential in assisting and improving nursing. AI offers ways to reduce costs and increase the efficiency of nursing. Despite the positive potential of AI, the complex ethical concerns of its introducting into nursing should be considered explicitly. Future research should also explore nurses' attitudes towards AI and their acceptance of AI technologies in the clinical setting.

Discuss the following questions with your partners.

1. What do you think about applying AI-based technologies in nursing?
2. Is it feasible to adopt Automated Screening of Literature on Artificial Intelligence in Nursing?
3. What is the advantage of autonomous robotic applications?

Task 1 Learn the following general academic vocabulary.

available methodological acquisition administrative computational interaction justify registration validate dimension implement principal statistical summarize modify perspective expertise interval utilize comprehensive extraction reinforcement protocol qualitative

Beginning to read

Task 2　Now read the text.

Text A

Artificial Intelligence-based Technologies in Nursing: A Scoping Literature Review of the Evidence
Hanna von Gerich et al

1. Artificial intelligence (AI) is an umbrella term used to describe techniques developed to teach computers to mimic human-like cognitive functions like learning, reasoning, communicating and decision-making. AI can be defined as: "software (and possibly also hardware) systems designed by humans that, given a complex goal, act in the physical or digital dimension by perceiving their environment through data acquisition, interpreting the collected structured or unstructured data, reasoning on the knowledge, or processing the information, derived from this data and deciding the best action(s) to take to achieve the given goal".

2. The history of AI in nursing spans over four decades. First mentions in the Medline database go as far back as 1985, with the introduction of expert systems providing clinical decision support, followed by state-of the-art nurse scheduling models. From the beginning, challenges facing the adoption of AI for nursing have raised concerns, and the need to develop new perspectives on technology adoption and identifying barriers in technology acceptance among nurses is equally as relevant today. The amount of research around AI in medicine and health has grown rapidly during the last decade, and the recent popularity in introducing AI in nursing is easy to justify. Today's data-rich healthcare ecosystem(数据丰富的医疗生态系统) offers numerous possibilities for AI developers, and AI offers ways to reduce costs and increase the efficiency of health care services. To that end, it is estimated that by 2025, AI could create potential healthcare savings of $150 billion.

3. Introducing AI-based technologies into the nursing discipline has raised concerns and public discussion, with many fearing that technologies will replace human-to-human interaction, compromising the ethics of care, while others are worried that AI will replace nurses. Other major concerns revolve around the ethical use of these technologies, such as managing data bias and its use to train algorithms. Some of these fears could be alleviated by providing adequate information on AI for

the end users，understanding the current research on these technologies，and through transparent discussion（透明的讨论）regarding the ethics of AI in nursing. When developed and implemented thoughtfully and thoroughly，AI-based technologies in nursing should be easy and intuitive to use. Such technologies can relieve nurses of administrative tasks，allowing for the concentration of their efforts on the core of professional care. A necessary step towards the broader benefits of AI-based technologies for nursing is the identification of the domains（域识别）where they present actual added value to nursing.

4. Nurses，both as potential users of AI-based technologies and as experts of professional care，are in a key position to shape and lead the evolution of modern AI in nursing. Although nurses' clinical and research expertise can play a vital role in co-designing nursing-relevant technologies，their current level of involvement in the research and co-design of these technologies remains unclear. However，nurses have often been excluded in the early analysis，development，and design phases of precision medicine and AI，only included to contribute their expertise in the late phases of testing when it could be used earlier in the process. The lack of a common vocabulary and understanding between the experts in nursing and technological domains is further suggested to be a barrier for nurse involvement in AI research and co-design. By gathering the current research evidence on AI-based technologies in nursing，the gap in knowledge，standardized definitions，concepts，and theories for AI in nursing can be narrowed.

5. The aim of this scoping literature review is to synthesize the currently available state-of-the-art research in AI-based technologies applied in nursing practice. This scoping review 1）summarizes the types of available evidence，such as applications of AI in nursing and their evaluation，2）reviews the involvement of nurses in technological development and research，and 3）examines ethical discussions（道德讨论）in published research.

6. This scoping review included articles that describe the development，testing, implementation，clinical use or optimization of technologies utilizing AI in the clinical nursing context. Due to the wide scale of available technologies defined as AI and the exponentially growing interest to develop technologies using AI in nursing，a scoping review to summarize and disseminate the findings was conducted following the methodological framework proposed by Arksey and O'Malley that was later advanced by Levac et al,. This methodological framework consists of five stages：（1）identifying the research questions，（2）identifying relevant studies，（3）study selection，（4）charting the data（绘制数据图表），and（5）collating，summarizing and reporting the results.

7. A search was conducted in March 2021 using the following electronic databases：PubMed（MEDLINE）（生物医药文献服务检索系统），CINAHL（EBSCO）（护理学文献

资料库），Web of Science and IEEE（电子与电气工程师协会）Xplore from January 1st 2010 to March 24th 2021. This time period was selected due to the rapid development and advancement of nursing technologies utilizing AI during the 2010s. Peer-reviewed journal articles written in English were included. A comprehensive search strategy was developed and refined in collaboration with our research team, and a health science librarian was consulted. The search terms （title and abstract） were "nurse * ", "nursing" and 61 relevant terms related to technologies, methodologies and algorithms used in artificial intelligence and machine learning.

8. The included studies focused on developing or validating AI-based technologies to be used in nursing care. The studies were experimental or observational using qualitative（定性的）, quantitative（定量的）or mixed methods approaches. Articles required a clear description of the relationship with, and the potential impact on, nursing. For example, studies where the nurses in the research had tested the implementation in the clinical setting, or where the authors had made a connection to the uses of the suggested technology as it pertains to the scope of nursing practice, were included. Studies that focused on key phases within AI development and application—technology development, technology formation （testing）, technology implementation or operation phase—were included.

9. We excluded studies that were not relevant to nursing, non-experimental or non-observational, or were literature review articles. Studies that did not evaluate the AI-based technologies used in the study, as well as research targeted at technology used in nursing research and education, were also excluded. Further excluded studies covered nursing robots and nursing management. Nursing robots were defined using the ISO8373 definition："systems of mechanical, electrical, and control mechanisms used by trained operators in a professional health care（专业卫生保健）setting that perform tasks in direct interaction with patients, nurses, doctors, and other health care professionals and which can modify their behavior based on what they sense in their environment."

From International Journal of Nursing Studies，2022，127（3）

New words and expressions

mimic /ˈmɪmɪk/ *v*. to copy the way sb speaks, moves, behaves, etc. 模仿

alleviate /əˈliːvɪeɪt/ *v*. to make something less severe 减轻,缓解

disseminate /dɪˈsemɪneɪt/ *v*. cause to become widely known 散布,传播

validate /ˈvælɪdeɪt/ *v*. prove valid; show or confirm the validity of something 使生效

pertain /pəˈteɪn/ *v*. to exist or to apply in a particular situation or at a particular time
存在;适用

collate /kəˈleɪt/ *v*. to collect information together from different sources in order to

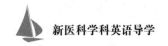

examine and compare it 核对

synthesize /ˈsɪnθəsaɪz/ *v*. combine so as to form a more complex，product 综合

thoroughly /ˈθʌrəli/ *adv*. in a complete and thorough manner 彻底地；完全地

intuitive /ɪnˈtjuːɪtɪv/ *adj*. spontaneously derived from or prompted by a natural tendency 直觉的

anomaly /əˈnɑməli/ *n*. deviation from the normal or common order or form or rule 异常

After reading

Task 3   Read Text A again and answer the following questions.

1. What is artificial intelligence?

2. Why is there growing concern about introducing AI-based technologies into the nursing discipline?

Task 4   Check your vocabulary. Fill in the blanks with the correct form of the words from the following box, each word can be used only once.

challenge(*n*.) import(*n*.) enable(*v*.) expert(*n*.) export(*n*.) fundamental
(*adj*.) diameter(*n*.) luxury(*n*.) tractor(*n*.) starve(*v*.) pollution(*n*.)
temporary(*adj*.) pest(*n*.)

1. To perform this analysis of CTL projects，DOE will need significant numbers of _____ staff members and additional equipment.

2. One reason stems from the increased use of mechanized technology，which replaces poor laborers who work for little，with _____ and other machinery.

3. These barriers are of particular _____ for youth with internalizing problems.

4. Monocultures of switch grass or other grasses provide few niches for natural predators that feed on crop _____ , so chemical pesticides are often applied.

5. Considering these aspects will continue to push nursing knowledge and practice further and will _____ nursing knowledge to be on par with other disciplines.

6. Recognition of perioperative stroke remains a major _____ .

7. More _____ parts of quality improvement are clinical trials and basic research to guide professionals toward which best practices need implementation.

8. Due to his COPD，his anteroposterior was greater than his transverse _____ .

9. The river parks would also filter air _____ and prevent soil erosion.

10. Merz Medizintechnik provided the software for data _____ of TEOAE measurements.

Task 5   Build your vocabulary. Read the sentences below, decide which word in each bracket is more suitable.

1. Air (blobs/bubbles) can appear as fluctuating small echoes.

2. Gene transcription is completed in different transcription (spots/sites).

3. BCL2 family members dictate cellular (fate/destiny) by regulating apoptosis.

4. They possess direct channels to (contact/communicate) with neighboring uterine SMC.

5. It has shown that hypoxia can create a/an (hostile/unfriendly) environment that promotes tumour growth.

6. Because possessions are so easily transferred, a remedy is required to safeguard them from (theft/burglary).

7. Sufficient mandates and funding should (urge/compel) DOE to implement efficiently.

8. Carcinoma specimen has been listed in the (brochure/catalogue) of Somatic Mutations in Cancer database.

9. This is achieved via a three-step (process/action) of selection, amplification, and characterization.

10. The constant anxiety of the trip becoming a bust has essentially (emptied/drained) much of the joy of the true experience.

Guiding to learn

Task 6   Learn the following general academic vocabulary.

assessment distribution formulate percentage variable appropriate relevance
consensus contribution maximum sequence validate dimension implement
parameter summarize marginal unstable explicit convert extract automate
qualitative

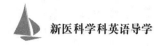

Beginning to read

Task 7　Now read the text.

Text B

Towards Automated Screening of Literature on Artificial Intelligence in Nursing
Hans Moen et al

1. Literature reviews are typically conducted for the purpose of summarizing existing scientific literature on a specific topic，or scientific field. The review type and methods depend on the research question at hand. One laborious phase of any literature review is the assessment of article relevance through screening and selection of articles （文章的筛选和选择）based on title and abstract. Research in nursing has increased exponentially during the last decade and almost 47,000 articles were indexed in PubMed in 2020 alone under（"Nursing"[MeSH] OR nursing）. The increasing need for evidence generation through evidence syntheses would benefit from technologies that reduce the manual labor required to conduct a literature review.

2. The use of machine learning methods in the form of natural language processing （NLP）（自然语言处理）and text classification has been shown to be promising when it comes to assisting the screening phase of literature reviews. For example，studies show that the specificity scores achieved by such NLP methods in systematic reviews in the field of medicine varies from 0.59 to 0.99. Approaches that have been explored include ensemble learning models（集成学习模型）；comparison of various machine learning algorithms for classification and comparison of different training set strategies；while several studies have evaluated the performance of off-the-shelf online machine learning and deep learning tools for semi-automated title and abstract screening.

3. In an ongoing study，we extracted 4,186 abstracts on the topic of "artificial intelligence （AI）in nursing" for manual screening（手动筛选）. Two reviewers manually screened these abstracts and found that 139（3.3%）should be included in the review. Given the rapid rate at which new literature is being published，we now would like to use the results from the previously conducted screening to train a text classification system that we can use to help us identify and suggest additional relevant articles that have not yet been manually screened. This includes articles that are published on the same topic in the future. The aim of this study is to evaluate the

applicability and performance of various text classification methods at the task of automated abstract screening on the research topic. The results could be useful for similar future efforts. Ethical review was not needed as the study was based on data published in scholarly journals.

Methods

Data

4. The data set used in this study contains 4,186 abstracts, out of which 139 (3.3%) were included. These abstracts were published after 2010 and were obtained from four databases: including PubMed (MEDLINE), CINAHL (EbSCO), Web of Science and IEEE. As search terms, we used a range of AI and machine learning methods and concept names combined with nursing specific terms. Database specific terms were also used when appropriate in the search. The abstracts were read and labelled independently by two domain experts to determine their eligibility for inclusion/exclusion based on the predefined criteria(预定义的标准). Disagreements were discussed until consensus was reached. Studies included were: experimental or observational studies; qualitative, quantitative and mixed methods approaches; and studies that developed or validated AI technologies applicable to nursing. Studies without explicit description of the relationship between the AI technology and potential impact on nursing practice or education were excluded.

BERT and BioBERT(生物医学语言模型)-Transformer-based language models

5. BERT is a popular transformer-based language model developed by Google. In this work, the biobert-v1.1 and the bert-base-uncased models were used via the Huggingface Transformers library. Combinations of values between $1\times10-1$ and $1\times10-15$ for both the learning rate and the epsilon parameter were evaluated. Model training was extremely unstable and the resulting F1-scores differed by even 20 percentage points on different runs with the exact same parameters, possibly due to the small dataset size. Thus, three duplicates were trained for each parameter combination, and the best model was chosen out of all the trained models based on development set performance.

BiLSTM(双向长短期记忆网络)-Bidirectional long short-term memory network

6. Long short-term memory (LSTM) (长短期记忆) network is a recurrent neural network architecture able to process sequential data (words in this case) in which each decision is influenced by the previous observations. Here we use bidirectional LSTMs, meaning the network reads the input sentence from both directions. As input layer we used an embedding layer initialized with pre-trained word embeddings. For the implementation we used the Keras API (应用程序接口), which runs on top of

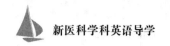

Tensorflow. Class weighting was used to tackle the data imbalance issue. Based on a simple grid search, the best performing model on the development set had two bidirectional LSTM layers, followed by three dense layers and finally the binary decision layer, all with Sigmoid activations.

CNN-Convolutional neural network

7. Convolutional neural networks (CNN)(卷积神经网络) for textual data treat each word in a sentence as a k-dimensional vector, after which convolution operations with various filters are applied to the concatenation. Sets of feature maps from the convolution operations are passed with maximum pooling to a fully connected Softmax layer whose output is the probability distribution over the labels to predict. The model was initiated with pre-trained word embeddings.

FastText-FastText classifier

8. FastText is a library for learning word embeddings and text classification created by Facebook Inc. It relies on a relatively simple densely connected neural network with the option to use n-gram features in addition to the individual words. To address the data imbalance issue, we here used an iterative method of oversampling(过采样迭代法). This implemented a random set of positive samples for each negative sample in the data set.

LinSVM-Linear support vector classifier

9. Support Vector Machine (SVM)(支持向量机) has been shown to be highly effective in classifying high-dimensional feature spaces such as vectorization of common words. This method was chosen because of its speed and simplicity in implementation. SVM works by iteratively finding the hyperplane(超平面) that separates two different classes with maximum marginal hyperplane and minimizing the error. SVM performance can be improved with stochastic gradient descent (SGD)(随机梯度下降) learning. Here we used SGD Classifier with Randomized search for choosing the optimal parameters.

RF-Random Forest

10. Random Forest (RF)(随机森林) is an ensemble of decision trees . It relies on a BoW representation of the text. Gradient Boosting Trees (GBT)(梯度提升树), which builds trees in a sequence based on the performance of the previous trees, were also tested. However, this did not give any improvements relative to RF.

LR-Logistic Regression with L1 and L2 constraints

11. Logistic regression models the probability of each abstract belonging to a

particular category based on their vectorized（向量化的）representations. Ridge regression（岭回归）minimizes regression coefficients for variables with minor contribution to the outcome. To convert the abstracts into a vectorized representation we used GloVe word embeddings. Oversampling was used to deal with the imbalanced data issue.

From Studies in Health Technology and Informatics，2022，290（6）

After reading

Task 8   Build your vocabulary.

Directions：Match the following words with their corresponding definitions and Chinese equivalents.

English：abstract   conduct   classification   consensus   duplicate   formulate   optimization   relevance

Chinese：摘要   执行   分类   共识   副本   构想   最优选   相关性

Paras. 1—7

English	Chinese	Definition
1. _____	_____	a. agreement in the judgment or opinion reached by a group as a whole
2. _____	_____	b. something additional of the same kind
3. _____	_____	c. the relation of something to the matter at hand
4. _____	_____	d. come up with（an idea, plan, explanation, theory, or principle）after a mental effort
5. _____	_____	e. to organize or do a particular activity
6. _____	_____	f. the act of rendering optimal
7. _____	_____	g. a short piece of writing containing the main ideas in a document
8. _____	_____	h. the act of distributing things into classes or categories of the same type

Paras. 8—11

English：embed   implement   maximum   previous   probability   regression   tackle

Chinese：嵌入   实施   最大极限的   先前的   可能性   退化   解决

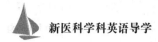

	English	Chinese	Definition

9. _____ _____ i. to make a determined effort to deal with a difficult problem or situation

10. _____ _____ j. the greatest or most complete or best possible

11. _____ _____ k. happening or existing before the event or object that you are talking about

12. _____ _____ l. how likely sth is to happen

13. _____ _____ m. to make sth that has been officially decided start to happen or be used

14. _____ _____ n. the process of going back to an earlier or less advanced form or state

15. _____ _____ o. to fix sth firmly into a substance or solid object

Guiding to learn

Task 9　Learn the following general academic vocabulary from the word bank.

> autonomous　eliminate　impair　eligible　behavioural　discrepancy
> methodological　agitation　agression　extensively　numerous　concurrently
> disruptive　qualitative　imperative　ducumentation

Beginning to read

Task 10　Now read the text.

Text C

Nursing Procedures for Advanced Dementia: Traditional Techniques Versus Autonomous Robotic Applications (Review)
Liliana David et al

1. Dementia（失智症）represents a major neurocognitive disorder caused by brain disease or injury and is characterized by impairments in executive function, learning and memory, attention, language, perceptual-motor function, and/or social

cognition, among other psychiatric, mood, and behavioural disturbances (行为障碍).

2. Unfortunately, the onset of this disease may be very subtle, and patients frequently present unspecific symptoms that can be easily confused with chronic fatigue syndrome(慢性疲劳综合征), depression, insomnia, anaemia, infections, side effects of medication, natural aging, nutrient imbalances, or vitamin and hormone deficiencies. For this reason, dementia is commonly misdiagnosed or overlooked in the earlier stages.

3. Since the average life expectancy has increased, dementia rates are rapidly growing in all continents. Epidemiologic studies (流行病学研究)revealed that ~6% of the population over 65 years is diagnosed with dementia, and 46.8 million people live with dementia worldwide. Furthermore, the total number of patients with dementia is estimated to double every 20 years. There is no curative treatment for the disease, and the burden on society is significant.

4. The main nursing interventions for patients with advanced dementia(晚期痴呆) include periodic change of position to avoid the appearance of pressure ulcers, active and passive mobilization, massage, passive feeding, skin hygiene, bed and body linen, bedding with flea(跳蚤) and urinary catheter management(导尿管管理). In the situation where these patients are immobilized in beds, it is necessary to prevent falls by properly arranging the space in the bed to eliminate safety risks. These procedures are used as an attempt to overcome complications of advanced dementia such as metabolic disorders related to nutritional deficiency, depression, selfinjury and impaired selfimage. Patients with advanced stages of dementia frequently require professional 24h supervision for their personal safety, basic needs, and the administration of medication. Autonomous robotic assistive technology (自动机器人辅助技术)may represent an affordable and practical solution to this global problem.

5. For this reason, the purpose of this study was to perform a comparative analysis of traditional nursing techniques and autonomous robotic applications used on patients with advanced stages of dementia.

6. PubMed, Cochrane Library, EMBASE, and WILEY data bases were searched for relevant articles regarding nursing techniques used in patients with advanced dementia, starting with traditional techniques and ending with artificial intelligence (AI)based systems and autonomous robots(自动机器人). The search terms included: (advanced dementia OR severe dementia) AND (AI OR robotic OR robots OR neural networks OR deep learning OR automated procedures OR autonomous application).

7. Exclusion criteria(排除标准) were: conference presentations, letters to the editor, studies written in languages other than English, case reports, pediatric studies, abstracts, and editorials (Fig. 1). A total of 2 independent authors (LD and SLP) reviewed eligibility titles, abstracts, and full text of eligible articles. Data extraction was conducted independently by both reviewers. Fig. 1 demonstrates the search

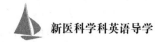

strategy using the PRISMA flow diagram(流程图).

8. Discrepancies related to the results of the quality assessment evaluation between the two investigators were resolved through discussion. Results of the methodological quality assessment did not have any effect on the eligibility of the studies in our systematic review.

9. Our search identified a total of 2,679 articles. Following use of human filters, the search identified 298 articles. Following application of all filters (human filters, while excluding conference abstracts and conference papers), 112 studies remained. Finally, a total of 23 articles were included in this systematic review: 8 studies analyzing traditional nursing techniques and 15 studies analyzing autonomous robotic applications.

Traditional nursing techniques for patients with advanced dementia

10. An extensive trial conducted by Husebo et al evaluated the effects of a 4 step pain management protocol on agitation, aggression, pain, activities of daily life, and cognition in patients suffering from moderate to severe dementia and clinically significant behavioural changes. All patients were residents of one of the 60 single independent nursing home units included in the trial. The outcome was evaluated using multiple measuring tools: CohenMansfield agitation inventory, neuropsychiatric inventory(神经精神量表)(nursing home version), mobilisation-observation-behaviourintensity-dementia-2 pain scale, activities of daily life, and Mini-Mental State Examination (MMSE). The active intervention proved to be of great benefit in addition to the non-specific effect, and the authors suggested that well-coordinated pain management could be used extensively for the assistance of agitated residents of nursing homes suffering from dementia.

11. Following performance of a systematic review of enteral tube feeding in patients with advanced dementia, Sampson et al concluded that the benefits are not supported by sufficient evidence despite numerous patients receiving this intervention. Concurrently, it appeared that the side effects of this procedure lacked adequate study.

12. A team led by Skovdahl et al studied the effect of tactile stimulation(触觉刺激) in five residents from a nursing home who suffered from behavioural and psychiatric symptoms of dementia. The caregivers were instructed on performing tactile stimulation and applied this technique at least once a week. Each session was documented using a form designed specifically for this purpose. The entire documentation containing 60 pages was then analyzed using qualitative content analysis. The sessions designed to continue for 28 weeks with a mean duration of 45 min had a positive and relaxing influence, however, the use of such therapies should be respectful towards the preferences of patients.

13. The effect of music therapy was studied by Ridder et al in an exploratory randomized controlled trial(探索性随机对照试验) that compared the standard care

group of patients with the groups receiving music therapy twice a week, for six weeks in a row. Music therapy demonstrated a positive effect on the quality of life and reduced agitation disruptiveness.

From Experimental and Therapeutic Medicine, *2022*, *23(2)*

New words and expressions

dementia /dɪˈmenʃə/ *n*. mental deterioration of organic or functional origin 痴呆症

impairment /ɪmˈpeəmənt/ *n*. the condition of being unable to perform as a consequence of physical or mental unfitness 障碍,损伤

eligible /ˈelɪdʒəbl/ *adj*. qualified for or allowed or worthy of being chosen 有资格的

filter /ˈfɪltə(r)/ *n*. a program that stops certain types of electronic information, email, etc. being sent to a computer 筛选程序

multifaceted /ˌmʌltɪˈfæsɪtɪd/ *adj*. having many aspects 多方面的

exhibit /ɪgˈzɪbɪtɪd/ *v*. to show clearly that you have or feel a particular feeling, quality or ability 表现出

conventional /kənˈvenʃənl/ *adj*. following what is traditional or the way sth has been done for a long time 传统的

apathy /ˈæpəθi/ *n*. the feeling of not being interested in or enthusiastic about anything 冷淡

extrapolation /ɪkˌstræpəˈleʃn/ *n*. an inference about the future (or about some hypothetical situation) based on known facts and observations 推断

agitation /ˌædʒɪˈteɪʃn/ *n*. a mental state of extreme emotional disturbance 焦虑不安

After reading

Task 11   **Build your vocabulary. Choose one word which can be used to replace the language shown in bold without changing the meaning of the sentence from the list below. Change forms and cases when necessary.**

bulk (*n*.)   fluid (*n*.)   fulfill (*v*.)   huge (*adj*.)   instance (*n*.)   inspect (*v*.)
novel (*n*.)   revolve (*v*.)   switch (*v*.)   shrunk (*v*.)   topic (*n*.)   vital (*adj*.)

1. The choice of an appropriate endpoint is **essential** for studies involving new therapeutic modalities.   _____

2. They went to extremes of exploitation in order to **keep** this perceived potential.   _____

3. We assessed adherence by **examining** blister packs for retained pills.   _____

4. If this sector slowly **change** over to renewable energy，the impact on the renewable energy market would be tremendous. _____

5. In looking at the variables we can use to move the **majority** of the atmospheric carbon to the deep oceans we have fixation，downwelling and deposition. _____

6. Disease experienced by His-panics in 1992 had **decreased** to 11% in 2012. _____

7. Currently，the first bolus began only for intravenous **liquid** administration documented as meeting bundle guidelines. _____

8. There were no **cases** of gross postoperative neurologic injury. _____

9. The dispute **rotates** around how land is used and how much influence local officials should have in managing those lands. _____

10. Such benefits could possibly be offset by **enormous** economic and environmental costs associated with the commercialization of GMOs. _____

Further reading

David，L.，Popa，S. L.，Barsan，M.，et al. (2022). Nursing Procedures for Advanced Dementia：Traditional Techniques versus Autonomous Robotic Applications (Review). *Experimental and Therapeutic Medicine*. 23(2).

Moen，H.，Alhuwail，D.，Björne，J.，et al. (2022). Towards Automated Screening of Literature on Artificial Intelligence in Nursing. *Studies in Health Technology and Informatics*. 290(6).

Mudgal，S. K.，Agarwal，R.，Chaturvedi，J.，et al. (2022). Real-world Application，Challenges and Implication of Artificial Intelligence in Healthcare：An Essay. *The Pan African Medical Journal*. 43(9).

Ronquillo，C. E.，Mitchell，J.，Alhuwail，D.，et al. (2022).The Untapped Potential of Nursing and Allied Health Data for Improved Representation of Social Determinants of Health and Intersectionality in Artificial Intelligence Applications：A Rapid Review. *Yearbook of Medical Informatics*. 31(1).

Von，Gerich，H.，Moen，H.，Block，L. J.，et al. (2022). Artificial Intelligence-based Technologies in Nursing：A Scoping Literature Review of the Evidence. *International Journal of Nursing Studies*. 127(3).